Helicobacter pylori - Diagnosis, Pathogenesis, and Treatment Strategies

Edited by Márcia Aparecida Sperança

Published in London, United Kingdom

Helicobacter pylori - Diagnosis, Pathogenesis, and Treatment Strategies
http://dx.doi.org/10.5772/intechopen.1008036
Edited by Márcia Aparecida Sperança

Contributors
Abdalrahman N. Herbawi, Abdul Qadir, Arti Wongcha-Um, Aychin I. Hasanova, Chuying Yu, Emin Kh. Verdiyev, Ferid V. Guliyev, Gulustan H. Babayeva, Gunay V. Asadova, Haoyu Zhao, Jamal S. Musayev, Kareem Ibraheem, Majed Dwaik, Nadeem Irshad, Nargiz E. Afandiyeva, Osama Hroub, Qingsheng Liu, Rafail H. Hasanov, Rashad A. Hasanov, Ratha-korn Vilaichone, Shahid Khan, Suting Qian, Tinpawee Thongkongthun, Umud R. Mahmudov, Varocha Mahachai, Xintong Ye

First published in London, United Kingdom, 2025 by IntechOpen
IntechOpen is the global imprint of INTECHOPEN LIMITED, registered in England and Wales, registration number: 11086078, 167-169 Great Portland Street, London, W1W 5PF, United Kingdom

For EU product safety concerns: IN TECH d.o.o., Prolaz Marije Krucifikse Kozulić 3, 51000 Rijeka, Croatia, info@intechopen.com or visit our website at intechopen.com.

British Library Cataloguing-in-Publication Data
A catalogue record for this book is available from the British Library

Helicobacter pylori - Diagnosis, Pathogenesis, and Treatment Strategies
Edited by Márcia Aparecida Sperança
p. cm.
Print ISBN 978-1-83635-349-2
Online ISBN 978-1-83635-348-5
eBook (PDF) ISBN 978-1-83635-350-8

If disposing of this product, please recycle the paper responsibly.

Meet the editor

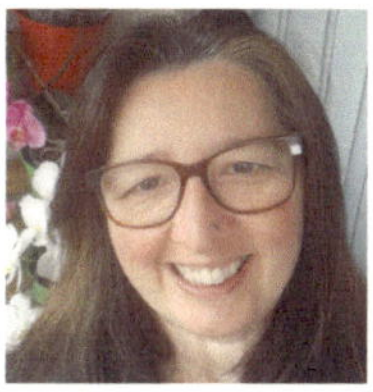

Márcia Aparecida Sperança is an Associate Professor at the Center for Natural and Human Sciences of Universidade Federal do ABC (UFABC, São Bernardo do Campo, São Paulo, Brazil). After obtaining a Ph.D. in Biology of Parasite-Host Interaction from the Parasitology Department of the Biomedical Institute of University of São Paulo (Brazil), Dr. Sperança worked as an Assistant Professor and Researcher at Marilia Medical School (Marília, São Paulo, Brazil). Her scientific experience is in diagnosis, molecular biology, and epidemiology of arboviruses, the bacteria *Helicobacter pylori*, malaria parasites, Chagas disease, leishmaniasis and COVID-19. Since 2009, Dr. Sperança is the head of the Laboratory of Pathogenic Agents at UFABC, an institution with multi and interdisciplinary academic proposals, which are characteristics of her investigation fields.

Contents

Preface

The Gram-negative, curved-shaped bacterium *Helicobacter pylori* was isolated from the gastric mucosal fragment of patients with gastritis in 1984 by two gastroenterologists, Marshall and Warren. Proof that *H. pylori* is responsible for causing gastric disease came from a rather bold experiment in which Barry Marshall himself ingested a solution containing the bacteria and, days later, developed gastritis. After receiving antibiotic treatment, he was cured, demonstrating the role of *H. pylori* in the genesis of gastric disease as an infectious agent. Since then, the treatment of ulcers and gastritis has been carried out with antibiotic therapy. The pathophysiology of gastric mucosal infection by *H. pylori* is associated with the genetic diversity of the bacteria, besides the immunological conditions and dietary habits of the human host. In addition to ulcers and gastritis, *H. pylori* is also classified as a Grade I etiological agent of gastric cancer by the World Health Organization. Since its discovery, the interactions of *H. pylori* with the gastric mucosa and its association with diseases have been investigated by several research groups worldwide. Thus, this book aimed to provide an update on the diagnosis, pathophysiology, and treatment of *H. pylori* in five chapters.

The first chapter, entitled "*Helicobacter pylori*: Etiology, Clinical Manifestations, and Advances in Treatment Strategies" is a revision about clinical manifestations and treatment strategies. The second chapter, entitled "*Helicobacter pylori*: Pathogenesis, Clinical Impact, and Modern Treatment Approaches" include in the revision, an update on mechanisms of bacterium pathogenesis. The diagnosis is included in chapter three, entitled "*Helicobacter pylori* Infection: Routine and Molecular Strategies for Diagnosing *Helicobacter pylori* in the New Era". Chapter four, entitled "Understanding Antibiotic Resistance Mechanisms in *H. pylori* and Its Clinical Implications", associates the mechanisms of *H. pylori* antibiotic resistance with clinical implications. The fifth chapter, entitled "*H. pylori* and Herpesviruses: "Commonwealth" or "Every Man for Himself" discusses the role of mucosa in immunity mechanisms and Herpesviruses and *H. pylori* infections, bilateral interferences in gastric mucosa alterations.

I am grateful to IntechOpen staff for the opportunity to participate as editor in this interesting book, with a high scientific level, contributing to several aspects of *H. pylori* associated with gastric diseases, and especially to Maja Bozicevic for her dedication and kind support as the manager in the publishing process. Also, I am grateful for the trust and precious contributions of all the authors of the chapters included in this book.

Márcia Aparecida Sperança
Centro de Ciâncias Naturais e Humanas,
Universidade Federal do ABC,
São Bernardo do Campo, São Paulo, Brazil

Chapter 1

Helicobacter pylori: Etiology, Clinical Manifestations, and Advances in Treatment Strategies

Shahid Khan, Abdul Qadir and Nadeem Irshad

Abstract

A common infection worldwide, *Helicobacter pylori* is a Gram-negative, microaerophilic bacterium that colonizes the gastric mucosa and is linked to gastric cancer, peptic ulcer disease (PUD), and chronic gastritis. Its epidemiology, which is fueled by fecal-oral or oral-oral transmission and made worse by inadequate sanitation, varies greatly across geographic and socioeconomic strata, with an estimated 50% global infection rate. Urease-mediated ammonia production, flagellar motility, and adhesins help the bacteria survive in the acidic gastric environment, while virulence factors like vacuolating cytotoxin A (VacA) and cytotoxin-associated gene A (CagA) cause inflammation, carcinogenesis, and damage to the epithelium. Clinical signs range from asymptomatic carriage to serious consequences, such as mucosa-associated lymphoid tissue (MALT) lymphoma and stomach adenocarcinoma, highlighting the importance of prompt identification. Improvements in invasive endoscopic techniques (histology, quick urease test) and diagnostic modalities (noninvasive urea breath tests (UBT), stool antigen assays (SAT), and serology) have increased the accuracy of detection. But increasing antibiotic resistance makes eradication less effective, requiring customized regimens such as vonoprazan-containing treatments, rifabutin-based protocols, and bismuth quadruple therapy. Resistance profiling and strain tracking are further made possible by molecular techniques such as fluorescence in situ hybridization (FISH) and next-generation sequencing (NGS). In order to maximize results, current guidelines place a strong emphasis on combination therapy, antimicrobial stewardship, and region-specific resistance trends. Promising approaches to reducing *H. pylori*-associated morbidity include host-microbe interaction research and novel approaches like probiotics, phytochemicals, and vaccine development. This chapter promotes interdisciplinary cooperation to address the ongoing worldwide burden by synthesizing recent discoveries on the pathogen's pathophysiology, diagnostic advancements, and changing therapy paradigms.

Keywords: *Helicobacter pylori*, gastric ulcer, peptic ulcer disease, antibiotic resistance, eradication therapy, gastric cancer, virulence factors, diagnostic methods

1. Introduction

The spiral-shaped, Gram-negative, microaerophilic *Helicobacter pylori* bacteria colonize the stomach mucosa and are linked to a number of gastrointestinal conditions, such as peptic ulcer disease, chronic gastritis, and gastric cancers. *H. pylori* has been identified as one of the most common bacterial illnesses since its identification in 1982 [1]. Clinical results vary greatly despite their widespread presence; some people experience serious problems such as mucosa-associated lymphoid tissue (MALT) lymphoma and stomach adenocarcinoma, while many people remain asymptomatic [2].

The bacterium's production of urease, which neutralizes gastric acid, and its motility, which permits it to pierce the protective mucus layer, give it the unusual ability to survive in the stomach's acidic environment [3]. Virulence factors that cause inflammation and damage to the stomach epithelium, such as vacuolating cytotoxin A (VacA) and cytotoxin-associated gene A (CagA), further contribute to the pathogenicity of *H. pylori* [4].

The fecal-oral or oral-oral route is the main method of transmission, and infections are usually contracted in childhood and, if left untreated, last a lifetime. Higher infection rates have been noted in underdeveloped nations, and socioeconomic factors, inadequate sanitation, and crowded living circumstances are important predictors of its prevalence [5, 6].

From minor dyspeptic symptoms to severe difficulties, the clinical presentation of *H. pylori* infection varies [7], requiring precise diagnostic techniques and efficient treatment plans. Detection rates have increased due to advancements in diagnostic procedures, including noninvasive tests like stool antigen and urea breath tests, as well as endoscopic biopsy-based treatments. However, eradication therapy is severely hampered by rising antibiotic resistance, which has led to the creation of innovative treatment plans [8, 9].

The pathogenesis, clinical signs, diagnostic methods, epidemiology, and current treatment recommendations of *H. pylori* infection are all thoroughly reviewed in this chapter. To minimize the worldwide burden of *H. pylori*-associated illnesses and optimize management techniques, a comprehensive understanding of this pathogen is necessary.

2. Epidemiology, transmission, pathogenesis, and clinical manifestations of *Helicobacter pylori* infection

2.1 Epidemiology

Helicobacter pylori infects nearly 50% of the global population, making it one of the most common bacterial infections. Its prevalence varies widely depending on geographic region, socioeconomic status, and hygiene practices. In developed countries, infection rates have dropped to 30–40%, largely due to improved sanitation and increased antibiotic use, while in developing nations, rates exceed 70%. Most infections occur in early childhood, but adults, particularly those traveling to high-prevalence areas such as military personnel, can also become infected [1, 10, 11]. Research by Vilaichone et al. highlights that prevalence not only differs between countries but can also vary significantly within different regions of the same nation [10].

2.2 Transmission

Although *H. pylori* transmission mechanisms are not fully understood, both direct (person-to-person) and indirect (environmental) routes are implicated [12].

In industrialized nations, interpersonal transmission dominates, whereas foodborne and waterborne spread prevails in regions with poor sanitation [13, 14]. Consumption of raw vegetables and exposure to contaminated water sources (e.g., streams, rivers) elevate infection risks, particularly in rural settings [15]. Despite limited evidence supporting foodborne environmental transmission, contaminated water remains a critical concern [13, 16].

Person-to-person transmission occurs via oral, fecal, or gastric routes [12]. The bacterium's presence in the saliva and dental plaque of infected individuals underscores its rapid spread, especially among families (**Figure 1**) [17–20].

2.3 Pathogenesis

Despite being primarily found in the stomach, *H. pylori* is surprisingly sensitive to hydrochloric acid solutions with a pH below 4.0 [21]. When *H. pylori* infections occur, there are four main components that contribute to the development of clinical illnesses such as ulcers and gastritis (**Figure 2**).

2.3.1 Urease activity

Helicobacter pylori survives the stomach's acidic environment (pH 4–6.5) despite not being acidophilic, adapting to transient acid shocks and thriving near pH 5.5 [22–24]. Initial theories suggested chemotactic motility toward the mucus layer via urea/bicarbonate gradients [25]. However, recent studies in gerbil models indicate pH gradients, not chemical cues, guide bacterial positioning in gastric mucus [26].

2.3.1.1 Urease-mediated acid resistance

Urease neutralizes acid by hydrolyzing urea into ammonia and bicarbonate, elevating local pH [27]. While all strains produce urease, its expression varies with

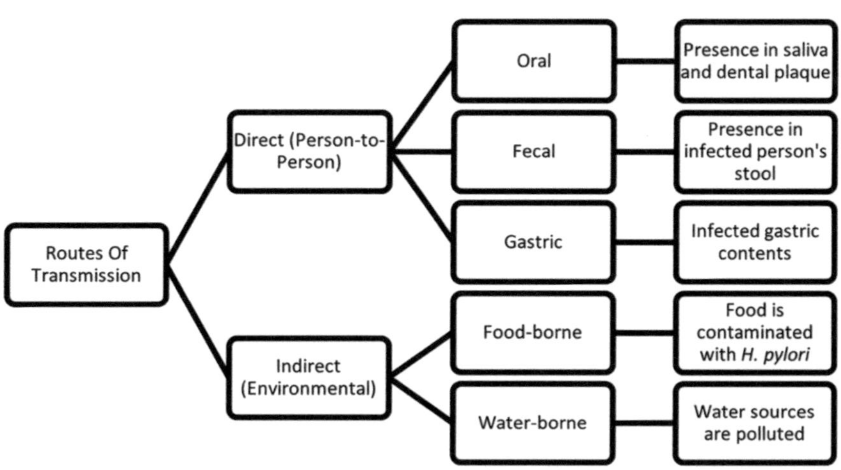

Figure 1.
Flowchart illustrating the transmission mechanisms of H. pylori, *categorized into direct (person-to-person) routes—including oral (via saliva and dental plaque), fecal (via infected stool), and gastric (via infected gastric contents)—and indirect (environmental) routes, such as food-borne (via contaminated food) and water-borne (via polluted water sources).*

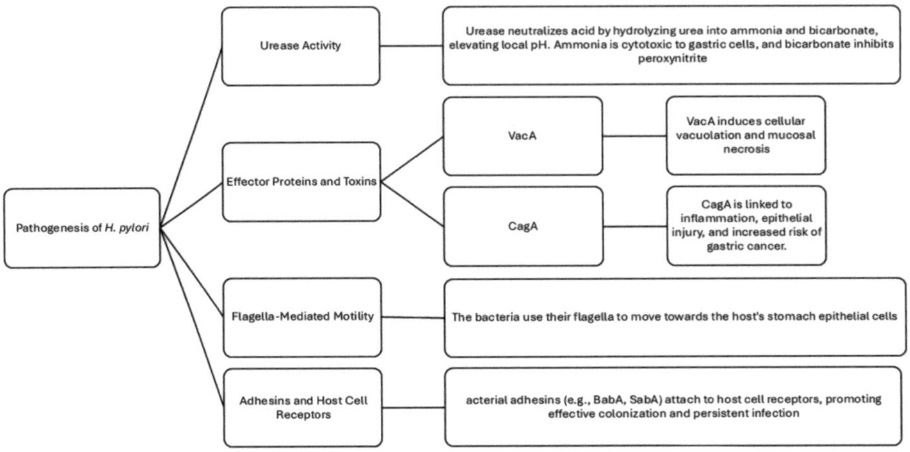

Figure 2.
Flowchart illustrating the key pathogenic mechanisms of H. pylori, *including urease activity, effector proteins and toxins (VacA and CagA toxins), flagella-mediated motility, and adhesion factors.*

environmental/strain factors [21, 28]. Early hypotheses proposed that outer membrane-associated urease neutralizes acid, but this mechanism is ineffective at very low pH [24, 29, 30]. Ammonia (cytotoxic to gastric cells) and bicarbonate (inhibits peroxynitrite) contribute to pathogenesis [31, 32]. Urease subunits (UreA/UreB) are potential therapeutic vaccine targets [33, 34].

2.3.1.2 Regulation of urease activity

Cytoplasmic urease activity is pH-dependent, with urea uptake controlled by the H^+-gated channel UreI [35–37].

$$(NH2)2CO + \mathrm{H2O} \rightarrow CO2 + 2NH3$$

2.3.2 Flagella-mediated motility

The bacteria travel toward the host's stomach epithelial cells via its flagella [38].

2.3.3 Adhesins and host cell receptors

By attaching themselves to host cell receptors, the bacterial adhesins (e.g., BabA, SabA) promote effective colonization and long-lasting infection [39].

2.3.4 Effector proteins and toxins

H. pylori damages host tissues via effector proteins like CagA (linked to inflammation, epithelial injury, and gastric cancer risk) and VacA (induces cellular vacuolation and mucosal necrosis). Infection triggers acute and chronic inflammation by activating eosinophils, neutrophils, mast cells, and dendritic cells. Gastric epithelial chemokines recruit neutrophils, exacerbating tissue damage and driving gastritis/ulcer formation. Chronic inflammation may progress to peptic ulcers, atrophic gastritis, or cancer, influenced by host genetics, immune responses, and environmental factors [40].

DOI: http://dx.doi.org/10.5772/intechopen.1010594

2.4 Clinical manifestations

Clinical signs of an *H. pylori* infection might range from asymptomatic colonization to severe gastrointestinal illness.

2.4.1 Asymptomatic carriage

The immune system keeps the infection under control but does not completely eradicate it, and the majority of infected people do not exhibit any symptoms [41].

2.4.2 Chronic gastritis

The most typical result is chronic inflammation of the stomach mucosa, which can eventually lead to atrophic gastritis [42].

2.4.3 Peptic ulcer disease (PUD)

Peptic ulcers: Responsible for >70% of gastric/duodenal ulcers, driven by bacterial toxin-induced mucosal damage and elevated acid secretion [42].

Gastric cancer: Classified as a Group I carcinogen (WHO) due to strong association with adenocarcinoma. Chronic inflammation triggers the Correa cascade (intestinal metaplasia → dysplasia → carcinoma) [42].

MALT lymphoma: Rare but aggressive; persistent infection drives B-cell proliferation. Eradication therapy induces remission in early stages [43].

Extragastric manifestations: Linked to iron-deficiency anemia, idiopathic thrombocytopenic purpura, and neurological disorders, though mechanisms remain unclear [44].

2.5 Diagnostic approaches

Accurate diagnosis is critical for *H. pylori* management. Methods are categorized as invasive (endoscopy-based tissue analysis) or noninvasive (detection of bacterial enzymes/antigens/DNA). Test selection depends on endoscopy necessity, cost, accessibility, patient age, and clinical context (initial vs. post-eradication) [45, 46]. **Figure 3** shows common *H. pylori* detection methods.

Key considerations:

Sensitivity/specificity: Critical for test accuracy and clinical decision-making [47].

Multi-testing strategy: Combining ≥2 high-accuracy tests enhances detection reliability [48, 49].

Understanding test limitations and performance metrics ensures precise diagnosis and effective management.

2.5.1 Noninvasive tests

2.5.1.1 Urea breath test (UBT)

The primary noninvasive method for detecting *H. pylori*. Utilizes ^{13}C (preferred, non-radioactive) or ^{14}C-labeled urea, hydrolyzed by bacterial urease into exhaled CO_2, measured 10 minutes post-ingestion [13, 34, 51–53]. **Figure 4** shows urea breath test diagrammatically.

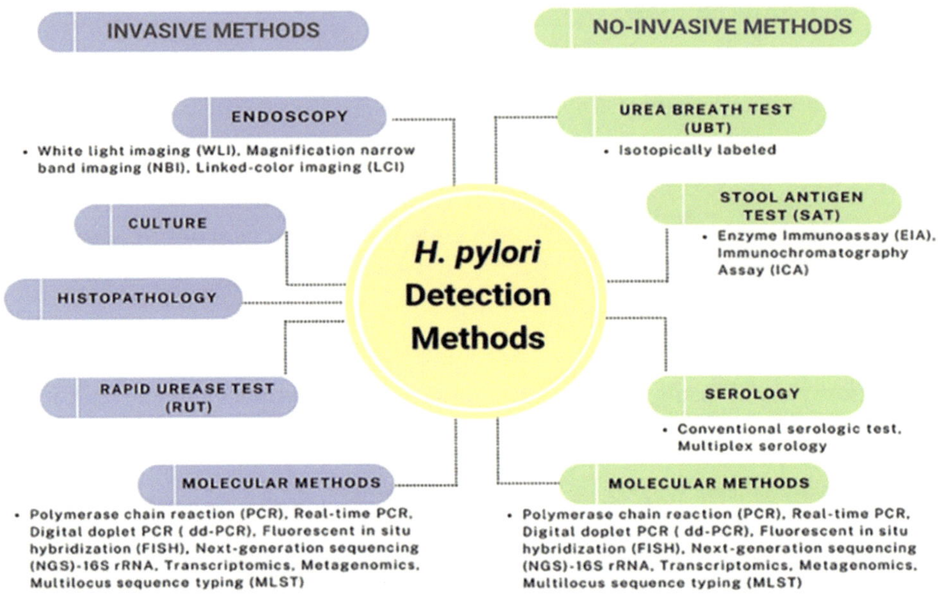

Figure 3.
H. pylori *detection Methods. Invasive methods include endoscopy, culture, histopathology, rapid urease test (RUT), and molecular techniques. Noninvasive methods include the urea breath test (UBT), stool antigen test (SAT), serology, and molecular techniques [50].*

Advantages:

High accuracy: >95% sensitivity/specificity in untreated patients without recent proton pump inhibitor (PPI)/antibiotic use [54].

Capsule-based ^{13}C-UBT: Reduces false positives from oral bacteria vs. liquid formulations [55].

Noninvasive: Cost-effective alternative in resource-limited settings [52].

Limitations:

False positives: Possible from non-*H. pylori* urease-producing bacteria (e.g., in hypochlorhydria) [52].

Protocol variability: Accuracy influenced by ^{13}C-urea dosage, breath collection timing (optimal at 20 minutes), and standardization [56, 57].

Clinical Superiority: Outperforms stool antigen/serology tests, particularly for eradication confirmation [56].

2.5.1.2 Stool antigen test (SAT)

Fecal samples can be evaluated for bacterial antigens using the Stool Antigen Test (SAT), which is appropriate for both initial diagnosis and post-treatment confirmation.

Types: Types include immunochromatography assay (ICA) and enzyme immunoassay (ELISA), which use either monoclonal or polyclonal antibodies (with monoclonal being favored for accuracy) [51, 59].

Advantages:

- No fasting or PPI discontinuation required (monoclonal antibodies) [51, 53].
- ICA offers rapid results, ideal for resource-limited settings [60].

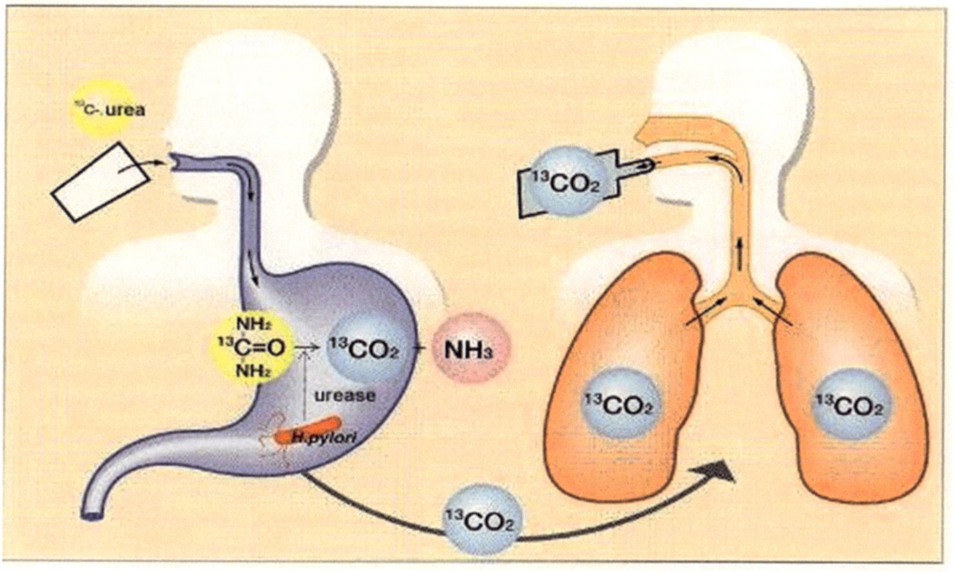

Figure 4.
Urea breath test for H. pylori *labeled urea is ingested; if* H. pylori *is present, urease breaks it down, releasing labeled CO_2, which is detected in the breath [58].*

- ELISA-based SAT serves as a reliable alternative to ^{13}C-UBT when validated with monoclonal antibodies [61].

Performance: Combining several tests increases diagnostic accuracy, and meta-analysis demonstrates constant sensitivity/specificity in children before and after treatment [53].

2.5.1.3 Serological testing

Targets: Detects IgG (most reliable), IgA, and IgM antibodies via EIA/ELISA/immunoblotting [62, 63].
Applications:

- *Initial screening for gastrointestinal bleeding, MALT lymphoma, or gastric cancer [64].*

- *High sensitivity/negative predictive value to exclude infection [64].*

- *Cost-effective dyspepsia screening in low-resource settings [8, 52].*

Limitations:

- *Cannot distinguish active vs. past infections (IgG persists post-treatment)* [62].

- *False positives in low-prevalence areas; requires region-specific validation* [65].

- *Reduced accuracy with urine/saliva samples* [62].

Advanced techniques:

Multiplex serology: Fluorescent bead-based detection of antibodies against 12–15 antigens for high-throughput risk stratification [66–68].

Key challenges:

- *IgG antibodies are detectable only ~ 21 days post-infection* [52].
- *Strain antigenic variability impacts test reliability* [65].
- *Limited utility of IgA/IgM tests due to lower accuracy and higher cost* [69].

Conclusion: Balances accessibility with the need for careful clinical interpretation and localized validation.

2.5.2 Invasive tests (endoscopic-based)

2.5.2.1 Histology

The gold standard for *H. pylori* diagnosis, histology combines direct visualization via staining (hematoxylin-eosin [H&E] or specialized methods like Genta stain/ immunohistochemistry) with high accuracy [70].

Procedure:

Biopsy protocol: Four mucosal samples (two from the gastric body, two from the antrum) optimize detection [71].

Staining:

Routine H&E: Sensitivity 70–95% [64].

Enhanced methods: Silver-based stains (e.g., Genta) or *H. pylori*.

Immunohistochemistry improves sensitivity [64].

Strengths:

Direct confirmation of infection and associated pathologies (e.g., gastritis, atrophy).

Limitations:

Accuracy is influenced by biopsy site (antrum/body), bacterial density, and interobserver variability [60].

Requires expert consensus for definitive diagnosis in ambiguous cases.

2.5.2.2 Rapid urease test (RUT)

The Rapid Urease Test (RUT) quickly detects *H. pylori* via urease activity in gastric biopsies [72]. It is a recommended first-line diagnostic when endoscopy is indicated [65]. The test involves placing the biopsy in a urea solution; urease produces ammonia and CO_2, raising pH and changing the indicator color. Biopsies from the antrum and body are recommended. False positives can occur from other bacteria [51], but oral urease has little effect due to denaturation [8]. The biopsy can be used for other tests, e.g., PCR [70].

2.5.2.3 Culture and antibiotic susceptibility testing

The culture method for detecting *H. pylori* is time-consuming and requires specialized conditions—such as cold temperature, microaerophilic environments, and enriched culture media [73]—limiting its use to specialized laboratories. It is primarily employed in scientific research or when previous treatments fail, as it enables customized therapy [51]. Less invasive alternatives, like gastric juice sampling or string testing, offer lower sensitivity compared to biopsy samples [8], and the quantity of detectable live *H. pylori* in gastric juice (median 1.75×10^1 cfu/mL) varies with disease severity, with not all organisms surviving in gastric fluid [74].

2.5.2.4 Molecular techniques (PCR)

When it comes to identifying antibiotic resistance mutations and non-culturable coccoid forms, molecular techniques improve the sensitivity of conventional diagnostic techniques for *H. pylori*. Essential methods consist of.

2.5.2.4.1 PCR-based methods

Target genes (vacA, cagA, 16S/23S rRNA, ureA, and glmM) in stomach biopsies, feces, or saliva are amplified by PCR variations (real-time, digital droplet, and nested). These methods offer excellent sensitivity but run the risk of false positives from nonspecific primers or dead bacterial DNA. To prevent cross-reactivity with related species, multi-gene analysis increases specificity [62].

2.5.2.4.2 Next-generation sequencing (NGS)

With 95–100% sensitivity for 16S rRNA amplicon sequencing, it permits thorough identification of virulence factors and resistance mutations (gyrA and 23S rRNA). Costly, unable to differentiate between live and dead germs, and possibly producing false positives are some of the drawbacks. Partial portions (e.g., V3–V4) do not have the same taxonomic resolution as full-length 16S rRNA sequencing (V1–V9 regions) [75].

2.5.2.4.3 Fluorescence In situ hybridization (FISH)

It finds the spatial distribution of *H. pylori* in biofilms and finds point mutations linked to resistance (such as clarithromycin), demonstrating excellent agreement with gold-standard techniques [76].

2.5.2.4.4 Multilocus sequence typing (MLST)

Seven conserved housekeeping genes are sequenced in order to monitor strain evolution, geographic origins, and mixed infections with heteroresistance, which refers to varying antibiotic susceptibility within a host, aiding in epidemiological research by supplementing whole-genome sequencing [77].

After therapy, PCR and NGS can produce misleading positive results due to residual DNA, which may complicate the assessment of treatment success. To address this and prevent inaccurate susceptibility findings, it is critical to test multiple biopsy samples from both the antrum and corpus regions, especially to detect heteroresistance [78]. While NGS and MLST offer promising avenues for personalized *H. pylori* treatment by tailoring approaches to individual infections, their widespread adoption is limited by high costs and the need for technical expertise. To ensure reliability, these molecular tools must be validated against conventional techniques [79].

2.6 Treatment and antibiotic resistance

The rising prevalence of antibiotic-resistant *H. pylori* strains has driven the evolution of treatment regimens. Current guidelines, notably the ACG Clinical Guideline, recommend eradication therapies tailored to local resistance patterns and informed by patient history, including past antibiotic exposure [80–82]. This approach ensures clinicians select effective treatments amidst growing resistance, emphasizing evidence-based, localized strategies to optimize outcomes.

2.6.1 Triple therapy

These medications serve as first-line treatments. **Table 1** shows the medications that are used in combination in triple drug therapy [82, 83].

2.6.2 Rifabutin-based therapy

When first-line medications do not work, rifabutin-based regimens are advised as rescue or salvage treatments [84]. **Table 2** shows medications which are used in rifabutin-based therapy.

2.6.3 Vonoprazan-based therapy

The following medications make up the first potassium-competitive acid blocker (PCAB)-based treatment that the FDA authorized in May 2022. For strains that are responsive to clarithromycin, it is an alternate first-line treatment [85]. **Table 3** shows medications which are used in vonoprazan-based therapy.

Drug with dosage	Duration	Success/eradication rate
PPI (e.g., omeprazole 20 mg BID, lansoprazole 30 mg BID, esomeprazole 40 mg QD, pantoprazole 40 mg QD, rabeprazole 20 mg BID) plus	14 days	14 days attain an *H. pylori* eradication rate of 81.9%, whereas 7 days attain an eradication rate of only 72.9%.
Clarithromycin 500 mg BID (clarithromycin resistance is less than 15%) or Metronidazole 500 mg BID (clarithromycin resistance is more than 15%) plus		
Amoxicillin 1000 mg BID or Metronidazole 500 mg BID (if not already selected)		

Table 1.
Drugs used in triple drug therapy.

Drug with dosage	Duration	Success/eradication rate
Amoxicillin 1 g every 8 hours plus	14 days	Based in part on the findings of two phase III trials that demonstrated eradication rates of 84.1% and 90.3%, the US Food and Drug Administration (FDA) authorized Talicia (a combination of three medications) for the treatment of *H. pylori* infection in 2019.
Omeprazole 40 mg every 8 hours plus		
Rifabutin 50 mg every 8 hours		

Table 2.
Rifabutin-based therapy drugs.

DOI: http://dx.doi.org/10.5772/intechopen.1010594

Drug with dosage	Duration	Success/eradication rate
Vonoprazan (PCAB) 20 mg BID plus	14 days	Similar to triple therapy
Amoxicillin 1000 mg BID plus		
Clarithromycin 500 mg BID		

Table 3.
Vonoprazan-based therapy.

2.6.4 Non-bismuth quadruple therapy

It is possible to provide non-bismuth quadruple (four medication) treatment concurrently or sequentially [82].

2.6.4.1 Sequential therapy

Sequential treatment for *H. pylori* involves taking drugs in a specific order: phase one with amoxicillin and a PPI for 5–7 days to reduce bacterial burden, followed by phase two with the same PPI plus metronidazole and clarithromycin for another 5–7 days to eliminate remaining germs [86]. **Table 4** shows medications which are used in sequential therapy.

2.6.4.2 Concomitant therapy

Concomitant treatment for *H. pylori* combines metronidazole, amoxicillin, clarithromycin, and a proton pump inhibitor (PPI), taken simultaneously for 10 to 14 days. This multi-drug strategy boosts eradication rates, curbs resistance, and excels against clarithromycin-resistant strains, with 14-day regimens achieving cure rates of at least 90%, outperforming standard triple therapy [87]. **Table 5** shows medications which are used in concomitant therapy.

2.6.5 Hybrid therapy

Sequential and concurrent therapy are combined in hybrid therapy. Since high percentages of eradication may still be obtained with various regimen lengths, 12 days is the ideal duration for hybrid treatment [88, 89]. **Table 6** shows medications which are used in hybrid therapy.

Drug with dosage	Duration	Success/eradication rate
PPI (e.g., pantoprazole 40 mg BID) plus Amoxicillin 1 g BID, then	5 to 7 days	14 days: 90.7–92.5% eradication rates. 10 days: 87% eradication rate.
PPI (e.g., pantoprazole 40 mg BID) plus Clarithromycin 500 mg BID or Tetracycline 500 mg QID	Next 5 to 7 dates (Total 10 or 14 days)	

Table 4.
Non-bismuth quadruple therapy: Sequential therapy drugs.

Drug with dosage	Duration	Success/ eradication rate
PPI (e.g., omeprazole 20 mg BID, lansoprazole 30 mg BID, esomeprazole 40 mg QD, pantoprazole 40 mg QD, rabeprazole 20 mg BID) plus	10 to 14 days	More than 90%
Amoxicillin 1000 mg BID plus		
Clarithromycin (1 g modified-release tablet QD or 500 mg BID) plus		
Metronidazole (500 mg TID)		

Table 5.
Non-bismuth quadruple therapy: Concomitant therapy drugs.

Drug with dosage	Duration	Success/eradication rate
PPI (e.g., pantoprazole 40 mg BID) plus Amoxicillin 1 g BID then	For 3 to 7 days	10-day: 95% 12-day: 95.1% 14-day: 93.4%
PPI (e.g., pantoprazole 40 mg BID) plus Amoxicillin 1 g BID plus Clarithromycin (1 g modified-release tablet QD or 500 mg BID) plus Metronidazole (500 mg TID)	For the next 7 days	

Table 6.
Hybrid therapy drugs.

2.6.6 Reverse hybrid therapy

Using the same medications as hybrid therapy but in the opposite order, as indicated in the accompanying table, reverse hybrid therapy combines sequential and concurrent treatment. Twelve days of reverse hybrid therapy yielded an eradication rate of 95.7%, which is comparable to that of 12 days of hybrid therapy (95.1 and 95.7%, respectively) [88, 89]. **Table 7** shows medications which are used in reverse hybrid therapy.

Drug with dosage	Duration	Success/eradication rate
PPI (e.g., pantoprazole 40 mg BID) plus Amoxicillin 1 g BID plus Clarithromycin (1 g modified-release tablet QD or 500 mg BID) plus Metronidazole (500 mg TID), then	7 days	12 days: 95.7%
PPI (e.g., pantoprazole 40 mg BID) plus Amoxicillin 1 g BID	For the next 3 to 7 days	

Table 7.
Reverse hybrid therapy drugs.

2.6.7 Bismuth-based therapy

An alternate first-line or second-line treatment is bismuth-based therapy (in regions with high levels of metronidazole and clarithromycin resistance, as well as in patients who have previously been exposed to macrolides or who are allergic to penicillin) [90]. **Table 8** shows medications which are used in bismuth-based therapy.

2.6.8 Regimen for high antibiotic resistance

In a population with a high level of antibiotic resistance, a team of Chinese researchers found that the concurrent treatment comprising levofloxacin and bismuth also produced good eradication rates [91]. **Table 9** shows regimen for high antibiotic resistance.

2.7 Medications with important clinical points

Clear instructions on how to take drugs, including knowing the recommended dosage, how to take them, and any considerations, must be given to patients. While combination medicine products should include pertinent information from the label, special counseling points can be given for medications. For clarity and simplicity of comprehension, several essential facts might be included in patient labeling [92]. **Table 10** shows medications with important clinical points.

Drug with dosage	Duration	Success/eradication rate
PPI or H2 receptor antagonist (e.g., lansoprazole 30 mg BID or famotidine 20 mg BID) plus	10–14 days	For 10 days: 90.4% For 14 days: 97.1%
Bismuth subsalicylate 525 mg QID or bismuth tripotassium dicitrate 300 mg QID plus		
Metronidazole 250 mg QID or 500 mg TID (or levofloxacin 500 mg QD) plus		
Tetracycline 500 mg QID		

Table 8.
Bismuth-based therapy drugs.

Drug with dosage	Duration	Success/eradication rate
Esomeprazole 20 mg BID plus	14 days	With Amoxicillin: 83.5% With cefuroxime: 81%
Levofloxacin 500 mg BID plus		
Bismuth 220 mg BID plus		
Amoxicillin 1000 mg BID or cefuroxime 500 mg BID		

Table 9.
Regimen for high antibiotic resistance.

Medicines	Important clinical points
PPI (Esomeprazole, Omeprazole, and Vonoprazan, etc.)	• Encourage the patient to report any systemic or cutaneous lupus erythematosus symptoms. • Tell the patient who has been taking many daily doses for more than a year to report any hip, wrist, or spine fractures that may be caused by osteoporosis. • Advise the patient to report any acute interstitial nephritis symptoms. • Before using antidiarrheal medication, advise the patient to see a healthcare provider and report any diarrhea that does not go away. • In addition to respiratory system problems and fever in children, side effects might include headache, nausea, vomiting, diarrhea, flatulence, and stomach discomfort in both adults and children. • Advise the patient to report any hypokalemia, hypocalcemia, or hypomagnesemia symptoms. • Advise the patient not to take St. John's wort while using this medication. • Encourage the patient to take the contents whole or to sprinkle them over a tablespoon of soft food. Do not chew the combination; instead, swallow it right away. Do not save it for later use.
Clarithromycin	• Encourage patients to report any signs of diarrhea linked to Clostridium difficile right away. • Because the medicine may produce dizziness, vertigo, confusion, and disorientation, warn the patient not to engage in activities that require mental attention or coordination until the effects are felt. • Abdominal discomfort, nausea, vomiting, and dysgeusia are possible side effects. • Tell the patient to eat before taking extended-release pills.
Metronidazole	• Advise patients to report any neurological problems right away. • Seizures, nausea, diarrhea, migraines, lightheadedness, metallic taste, rash, pruritus, or moderate leukopenia are possible side effects. • Recommend that the patient take the extended-release pill at least one hour before or two hours after eating. • During treatment and for three days after it, advise the patient to abstain from alcohol and propylene glycol-containing items since they might increase systemic exposure and have negative consequences.
Amoxicillin	• Advise the patient to stop taking the medication and to report any signs of a serious cutaneous adverse response, such as mucosal lesions or skin rash, right away. • Before using antidiarrheal medication, advise the patient to notify a healthcare provider if they have severe diarrhea. • A vulvovaginal mycotic infection, headache, nausea, and vomiting are possible side effects. • At around the same time each day, and within an hour after finishing a meal, advise the patient to take their medication.

DOI: http://dx.doi.org/10.5772/intechopen.1010594

Medicines	Important clinical points
Rifabutin	• Encourage patients to report symptoms of active TB or mycobacterium avium complex illness (MAC). • Advise patients to report severe cutaneous adverse effects, such as Stevens-Johnson syndrome, toxic epidermal necrolysis, drug response with eosinophilia and systemic symptoms (DRESS), or acute widespread exanthematous pustulosis. • Warn the patient that the medicine may produce brown-orange staining of fluids/tissues (skin, urine, feces, sputum, tears, and perspiration), which can irreversibly stain soft contact lenses. • Rash, stomach discomfort, nausea, taste perversion, and dyspepsia are among the possible side effects. • Advise the patient to report severe diarrhea and see a healthcare expert before taking antidiarrheal medications. • Advise patients who experience nausea, vomiting, or gastrointestinal disturbance to take the medicine with meals.
Tetracycline	• The drug induces sun sensitivity. Advise the patient to use sunscreen and avoid tanning beds. • Warn the patient that concurrent use of this medication may reduce the efficacy of oral contraceptives. Recommend an extra method of birth control. • The medication may induce diarrhea, nausea, and vomiting. • Patients should take the medication one hour before or two hours after meals. • Advise patients to avoid taking the medicine with milk or dairy products, as they may interfere with absorption. • Patients should avoid taking iron-containing preparations, as well as aluminum-, calcium-, and magnesium-containing antacids or supplements, since they might interfere with tetracycline absorption.
Bismuth	• Do not give the drug to children or teens with viral illnesses or chickenpox symptoms. • Warn patients that the medicine may produce brief, harmless darkening of the tongue and/or stool. • This medication might induce constipation, diarrhea, nausea, or vomiting. • Instruct patients to report indications of neurotoxicity, especially while taking high dosages of the medicine.

Medicines	Important clinical points
Levofloxacin	• Instruct patients to report any symptoms of tendonitis, tendon rupture, or peripheral neuropathy. • Advise patients to report symptoms of aortic aneurysm and dissection (e.g., abrupt chest, stomach, or back discomfort). • Advise patients to apply sunscreen, wear protective clothes, and avoid tanning beds to prevent photosensitivity. • Advise patients to avoid tasks that require mental alertness or coordination until the drug's effects are felt, since it may induce adverse effects on the central nervous system (e.g. dizziness, lightheadedness, elevated intracranial pressure). • Instruct patients to report any symptoms of hepatotoxicity promptly. • Possible side effects include nausea, headaches, sleeplessness, and constipation. • Ophthalmic side effects may include reduced or impaired vision. • Encourage patients to report symptoms of QT prolongation or recurrent diarrhea. • Instruct diabetic patients to report signs of insufficient glycemic control and recommend more regular blood glucose testing. • Advise patients to take oral solution 1 hour before or 2 hours after meals. • Instruct patients to take oral medication at the same time every day, with plenty of water. • Instruct patients to take oral medication 2 hours before or after magnesium or aluminum antacids, sucralfate, didanosine (buffered tablets or powder for oral solution), or iron or zinc preparations.
Cefuroxime	• Advise patients to see a healthcare practitioner if they experience watery and bloody stools (with or without stomach pains and fever) even after 2 months of medication therapy. • The drug can induce thrombophlebitis, diarrhea, nausea, rash, pruritus, urticaria, and vaginitis (including vaginal candidiasis). • Warn women taking combination estrogen and progesterone oral contraceptives that effectiveness may decrease.
Misoprostol	• Female patients should avoid pregnancy throughout medication and for at least a month following cessation. • Possible side effects include stomach discomfort, diarrhea, dyspepsia, flatulence, nausea, vomiting, and headache. • Advise patients to consume with meals to reduce gastrointestinal discomfort. • Warn patients to avoid using nonprescription magnesium-containing antacids, since these may increase the risk of diarrhea.

Table 10.
Medications with important clinical points.

DOI: http://dx.doi.org/10.5772/intechopen.1010594

3. Conclusions

Helicobacter pylori remains a significant global health threat, linked to peptic ulcers, chronic gastritis, and gastric malignancies, particularly in resource-limited regions. Its survival in acidic environments, aided by virulence factors like CagA and VacA, drives asymptomatic yet progressive damage. While noninvasive diagnostics (e.g., urea breath tests, stool antigen assays) improve detection, rising antibiotic resistance challenges eradication. Current therapies prioritize bismuth quadruple regimens, rifabutin-based protocols, and vonoprazan, with tailored approaches guided by susceptibility testing. Future strategies hinge on vaccine development and host-directed therapies. Combating *H. pylori* requires multidisciplinary collaboration—integrating public health initiatives, antimicrobial stewardship, and clinician education—to enhance early diagnosis, optimize treatments, and reduce global disease burden.

Author details

Shahid Khan, Abdul Qadir and Nadeem Irshad*
Department of Pharmacy, Quaid-i-Azam University, Islamabad, Pakistan

*Address all correspondence to: nirshad@qau.edu.pk

References

[1] Clarke E. *Helicobacter pylori*: A comprehensive review of pathogenesis, epidemiology, diagnosis, and therapeutic strategies. Insight into Epidemiology. 2024;**1**(1)

[2] Laszewicz W, Iwańczak F, Iwańczak B. Seroprevalence of *Helicobacter pylori* infection in polish children and adults depending on socioeconomic status and living conditions. Advances in Medical Sciences. 2014;**59**:147150. DOI: 10.1016/j.advms.2014.01.003

[3] Lee JH, Jun SH, Kim JM, Baik SC, Lee JC. Morphological changes in human gastric epithelial cells induced by nuclear targeting of *Helicobacter pylori* urease subunit a. Journal of Microbiology. 2015;**53**:406-414

[4] Amieva MR, El-Omar EM. Host-bacterial interactions in *Helicobacter pylori* infection. Gastroenterology. 2008;**134**:306-323. DOI: 10.1053/j.gastro.2007.11.009

[5] Ceylan A, Kirimi E, Tuncer O, Türkdoğan K, Ariyuca S, Ceylan N. Prevalence of *Helicobacter pylori* in children and their family members in a district in Turkey. Journal of Health, Population, and Nutrition. 2007;**25**(4):422-427

[6] Brown LM. *Helicobacter pylori*: Epidemiology and routes of transmission. Epidemiologic Reviews. 2000;**22**:283-297. DOI: 10.1093/oxfordjournals.epirev.a018040

[7] Sugano K, Tack J, Kuipers EJ, et al. For the faculty members of Kyoto global consensus conference. Kyoto global consensus report on *Helicobacter pylori* gastritis. Gut. 2015;**64**(9):1353-1367

[8] Garza-González E, Perez-Perez GI, Maldonado-Garza HJ, Bosques-Padilla FJ. A review of *Helicobacter pylori* diagnosis, treatment, and methods to detect eradication. World Journal of Gastroenterology. 2014;**20**:1438-1449. DOI: 10.3748/wjg. v20.i6.1438

[9] Pohl D, Keller PM, Bordier V, Wagner K. Review of current diagnostic methods and advances in *Helicobacter pylori* diagnostics in the era of next generation sequencing. World Journal of Gastroenterology. 2019;**25**:4629-4660. DOI: 10.3748/wjg.v25.i32.4629

[10] Vilaichone R-K, Mahachai V, Shiota S, Uchida T, Ratanachu-ek T, Tshering L, et al. Extremely high prevalence of *Helicobacter pylori* infection in Bhutan. World Journal of Gastroenterology. 2013;**19**:2806-2810. DOI: 10.3748/wjg.v19.i18.2806

[11] Magalhães Queiroz DM, Luzza F. Epidemiology of *Helicobacter pylori* infection. Helicobacter. 2006;**11**:1-5

[12] Zamani M, Vahedi A, Maghdouri Z, shokri-shirvani J. Role of food in environmental transmission of *Helicobacter pylori*. Caspian Journal of Internal Medicine. 2017;**8**:146-152. DOI: 10.22088/cjim.8.3.146

[13] Vale FF, Vítor JMB. Transmission pathway of *Helicobacter pylori*: Does food play a role in rural and urban areas? International Journal of Food Microbiology. 2010;**138**:1-12. DOI: 10.1016/j.ijfoodmicro.2010.01.016

[14] Zhang YY, Xia HH, Zhuang ZH, Zhong J. Review article: 'True' re-infection of *Helicobacter pylori* after successful eradication—worldwide annual rates, risk factors and clinical

implications. Alimentary Pharmacology & Therapeutics. 2009;**29**:145-160. DOI: 10.1111/j.1365-2036.2008.03873.x

[15] Cover TL, Blaser MJ. Helicobacter pylori and other gastric helicobacter species. In: Mandell, Douglas, and Bennett's Principles and Practice of Infectious Diseases. Philadelphia, Pennsylvania: Elsevier Inc.; 2014

[16] Quaglia NC, Dambrosio A. *Helicobacter pylori*: A foodborne pathogen? World Journal of Gastroenterology. 2018;**24**:3472-3487. DOI: 10.3748/wjg.v24.i31.3472

[17] Nisha KJ, Nandakumar K, Shenoy KT, Janam P. Periodontal disease and *Helicobacter pylori* infection: A community-based study using serology and rapid urease test. Journal of Investigative and Clinical Dentistry. 2016;7:37-45. DOI: 10.1111/jicd.12122

[18] Aksit BD, Akyuz S, Kıratlı B, Usta M, Urganci N, Alev B, et al. The investigation of *Helicobacter pylori* in the dental biofilm and saliva samples of children with dyspeptic complaints. BMC Oral Health. 2017;**17**:67. DOI: 10.1186/s12903-017-0361-x

[19] Silva DG, Stevens RH, Macedo JM, Albano RM, Falabella ME, Fischer RG, et al. Presence of *Helicobacter pylori* in supragingival dental plaque of individuals with periodontal disease and upper gastric diseases. Archives of Oral Biology. 2010;**55**:896-901. DOI: 10.1016/j.archoralbio.2010.06.018

[20] Goh KL, Chan WK, Shiota S, Yamaoka Y. Epidemiology of *Helicobacter pylori* infection and public health implications. Helicobacter. 2011;**16**:1-9. DOI: 10.1111/j.1523-5378.2011.00874.x

[21] Kusters JG, van Vliet AH, Kuipers EJ. Pathogenesis of *Helicobacter pylori* infection. Clinical Microbiology Reviews. 2006;**19**:449-490

[22] Schade C, Flemstrom G, Holm L. Hydrogen ion concentration in the mucus layer on top of acid-stimulated and -inhibited rat gastric mucosa. Gastroenterology. 1994;**107**:180-188

[23] Bijlsma JJ, Lie-A-Ling M, Nootenboom IC, Vandenbroucke-Grauls CM, Kusters JG. Identification of loci essential for the growth of *Helicobacter pylori* under acidic conditions. The Journal of Infectious Diseases. Nov 2000;**182**(5):1566-1569. DOI: 10.1086/315855. Epub 2000 Oct 9

[24] Stingl K, Altendorf K, Bakker EP. Acid survival of *Helicobacter pylori*: How does urease activity trigger cytoplasmic pH homeostasis? Trends in Microbiology. 2002;**10**:70-74

[25] Schreiber S, Bucker R, Groll C, Azevedo-Vethacke M, Garten D, Scheid P, et al. Rapid loss of motility of *Helicobacter pylori* in the gastric lumen *in vivo*. Infection and Immunity. 2005;**73**:1584-1589

[26] Schreiber S, Konradt M, Groll C, Scheid P, Hanauer G, Werling HO, et al. The spatial orientation of *Helicobacter pylori* in the gastric mucus. Proceedings of the National Academy of Sciences of the United States of America. 2004;**101**:5024-5029

[27] Burne RA, Chen YM. Bacterial ureases in infectious diseases. Microbes and Infection. 2000;**2**:533-542

[28] Contreras M, Thiberge JM, Mandrand-Berthelot MA, Labigne A. Characterization of the roles of NikR, a nickel-responsive pleiotropic autoregulator of *Helicobacter pylori*. Molecular Microbiology. 2003;**49**:947-963

[29] Sachs G, Scott D, Weeks D, Melchers K. The compartment buffered by the urease of *Helicobacter pylori*: Cytoplasm or periplasm? Trends in Microbiology. 2002;**10**:217-218

[30] Ha NC, Oh ST, Sung JY, Cha KA, Lee MH, Oh BH. Supramolecular assembly and acid resistance of *Helicobacter pylori* urease. Nature Structural Biology. 2001;**8**:505-509

[31] Smoot DT, Mobley HL, Chippendale GR, Lewison JF, Resau JH. *Helicobacter pylori* urease activity is toxic to human gastric epithelial cells. Infection and Immunity. 1990;**58**:1992-1994

[32] Kyriazanos LD, Ilias L, Gizaris V, Hountis P, Georgaklis V, Dafnopoulou A, et al. Seroepidemiology of *Helicobacter pylori* infection in Hellenic navy recruits. European Journal of Epidemiology. 2001;**17**:501-504

[33] Nomura S, Suzuki H, Masaoka T, Kurabayashi K, Ishii H, Kitajima M, et al. Effect of dietary anti-urease immunoglobulin Y on *Helicobacter pylori* infection in Mongolian gerbils. Helicobacter. 2005;**10**:43-52

[34] Velin D, Bachmann D, Bouzourene H, Michetti P. Mast cells are critical mediators of vaccine-induced *Helicobacter* clearance in the mouse model. Gastroenterology. 2005;**129**:142-155

[35] Weeks DL, Eskandari S, Scott DR, Sachs G. A H+-gated urea channel: The link between *Helicobacter pylori* urease and gastric colonization. Science. 2000;**287**:482-485

[36] Scott DR, Marcus EA, Weeks DL, Lee A, Melchers K, Sachs G. Expression of the *Helicobacter pylori* ureI gene is required for acidic pH activation of cytoplasmic urease. Infection and Immunity. 2000;**68**:470-477

[37] Bury-Mone S, Skouloubris SS, Labigne A, De Reuse H. The *Helicobacter pylori* UreI protein: Role in adaptation to acidity and identification of residues essential for its activity and for acid activation. Molecular Microbiology. 2001;**42**:1021-1034

[38] Keilberg D, Ottemann KM. How *Helicobacter pylori* senses, targets and interacts with the gastric epithelium. Environmental Microbiology. 2016;**18**(3):791-806

[39] Vaca DJ, Thibau A, Schütz M, Kraiczy P, Happonen L, Malmström J, et al. Interaction with the host: The role of fibronectin and extracellular matrix proteins in the adhesion of gram-negative bacteria. Medical Microbiology and Immunology. 2020;**209**(3):277-299

[40] Chmiela M, Kupcinskas J. Pathogenesis of *Helicobacter pylori* infection. Helicobacter. 2019;**24**:e12638

[41] Janeway CA. How the immune system works to protect the host from infection: A personal view. Proceedings. National Academy of Sciences. United States of America. 2001;**98**(13):7461-7468. DOI: 10.1073/pnas.131202998

[42] Zhang C, Yamada N, Wu YL, Wen M, Matsuhisa T, Matsukura N. *Helicobacter pylori* infection, glandular atrophy and intestinal metaplasia in superficial gastritis, gastric erosion, erosive gastritis, gastric ulcer and early gastric cancer. World Journal of Gastroenterology: WJG. 2005;**11**(6):791

[43] Salar A. Gastric MALT lymphoma and *Helicobacter pylori*. Medicina Clínica (English Edition). 2019;**152**(2):65-71

[44] Wong F, Rayner-Hartley E, Byrne MF. Extra intestinal manifestations

of *Helicobacter pylori*: A concise review. World Journal of Gastroenterology: WJG. 2014;**20**(34):11950

[45] Malfertheiner P, Camargo MC, El-Omar E, Liou J-M, Peek R, Schulz C, et al. *Helicobacter pylori* infection. Nature Reviews. Disease Primers. 2023;**9**(1):19. DOI: 10.1038/s41572023-00431-8

[46] Cardos AI, Maghiar A, Zaha DC, Pop O, Fritea L, Miere (Groza) F, et al. Evolution of diagnostic methods for *Helicobacter pylori* infections: From traditional tests to high technology, advanced sensitivity and discrimination tools. Diagnostics. 2022;**12**(2):508. DOI: 10.3390/diagnostics12020508

[47] Shreffler J, Huecker MR. Diagnostic Testing Accuracy: Sensitivity, Specificity, Predictive Values and Likelihood Ratios. Treasure Island (FL): StatPearls Publishing; 2023

[48] Hibaoui L, Massik A, Lebbar Z, Yahyaoui G, Mahmoud M, Bougnouch L, et al. The high sensitivity and specificity of rapid urease test in diagnosis of *Helicobacter pylori* infection in Moroccan children. Iranian Journal of Microbiology. 2022;**14**(5):669-676. DOI: 10.18502/ijm.v14i5.10960

[49] Yang H, Hu B. Diagnosis of *Helicobacter pylori* infection and recent advances. Diagnostics. 2021;**11**(8):1305

[50] Costa LC, Carneiro M, et al. Diagnostic methods for *Helicobacter pylori*. Medical Principles and Practice. 2024;**33**:173-184. DOI: 10.1159/000538349

[51] Sabbagh P, Mohammadnia-Afrouzi M, Javanian M, Babazadeh A, Koppolu V, Vasigala VR, et al. Diagnostic methods for *Helicobacter pylori* infection: Ideals, options, and limitations. European Journal of Clinical Microbiology & Infectious Diseases. 2019;**38**(1):55-66. DOI: 10.1007/s10096-018-3414-4

[52] Miftahussurur M. Noninvasive *Helicobacter pylori* diagnostic methods in Indonesia. Gut Liver. 2020;**14**(5):553-559. DOI: 10.5009/gnl19264

[53] Coelho LGV, Marinho JR, Genta R, Ribeiro LT, Passos M, Zaterka S, et al. IVth Brazilian consensus conference on *Helicobacter pylori* infection. Arquivos de Gastroenterologia. 2018;**55**(2):97

[54] Mattar R, Villares CA, Marostegam PFF, Chaves CE, Pinto VB, Carrilho FJ. Low dose capsule based ^{13}C-urea breath test compared with the conventional ^{13}C-urea breath test and invasive tests. Arquivos de Gastroenterologia. 2014;**51**(2):133-138. DOI: 10.1590/s0004-28032014000200012

[55] Osaki T, Mabe K, Hanawa T, Kamiya S. Urease-positive bacteria in the stomach induce a false-positive reaction in a urea breath test for diagnosis of *Helicobacter pylori* infection. Journal of Medical Microbiology. 2008;**57**(Pt 7):814-819. DOI: 10.1099/jmm.0.47768-0

[56] Best L, Takwoingi Y, Siddique S, Selladurai A, Gandhi A, Low B, et al. Non-invasive diagnostic tests for *Helicobacter pylori* infection. Cochrane Database of Systematic Reviews. 2018;**2018**(3):CD012080. DOI: 10.1002/14651858.cd012080. pub2

[57] Abd Rahim MA, Johani FH, Shah SA, Hassan MR, Abdul Manaf MR. ^{13}C-urea breath test accuracy for *Helicobacter pylori* infection in the Asian population: A meta-analysis. Annals of Global Health. 2019;**85**(1):110. DOI: 10.5334/aogh.2570

[58] FV Hospital. Urea Breath Test Illustration [Image]. 2019. Available

from: https://www.fvhospital.com/wp-content/uploads/2019/05/urea-brea-breath-2.jpg

[59] Qiu E, Li Z, Han S. Methods for detection of *Helicobacter pylori* from stool sample: Current options and developments. Brazilian Journal of Microbiology. 2021;**52**(4):2057-2062. DOI: 10.1007/s42770021-00589-x

[60] Urgessa NA, Geethakumari P, Kampa P, Parchuri R, Bhandari R, Alnasser AR, et al. A comparison between histology and rapid urease test in the diagnosis of *Helicobacter pylori* in gastric biopsies: A systematic review. Cureus. 2023;**15**(5):e39360. DOI: 10.7759/cureus.39360

[61] Zhou X, Su J, Xu G, Zhang G. Accuracy of stool antigen test for the diagnosis of *Helicobacter pylori* infection in children: A meta analysis. Clinics and Research in Hepatology and Gastroenterology. 2014;**38**(5):629-638. DOI: 10.1016/j.clinre.2014.02.001

[62] Alihosseini S, Jaberinezhad M, Sadeghpour Heravi F, Ghotaslou R, Ebrahimzadeh Leylabadlo H. Invasive and noninvasive *Helicobacter pylori* diagnostic methods in Iran. Gene Reports. 2020;**20**:100749. DOI: 10.1016/j.genrep.2020.100749

[63] Michel A, Waterboer T, Kist M, Pawlita M. *Helicobacter pylori* multiplex serology. Helicobacter. 2009;**14**(6):525-535. DOI: 10.1111/j.1523-5378.2009.00723.x

[64] Bosch DE, Krumm N, Wener MH, Yeh MM, Truong CD, Reddi DM, et al. Serology is more sensitive than urea breath test or stool antigen for the initial diagnosis of *Helicobacter pylori* gastritis when compared with histopathology. American Journal of Clinical Pathology. 2020;**154**(2):255-265. DOI: 10.1093/ajcp/aqaa043

[65] Malfertheiner P, Megraud F, O'Morain CA, Gisbert JP, Kuipers EJ, Axon AT, et al. Management of *Helicobacter pylori* infection: The Maastricht V/Florence consensus report. Gut. 2017;**66**(1):6-30. DOI: 10.1136/gutjnl-2016-312288

[66] Yao P, Kartsonaki C, Butt J, Jeske R, de Martel C, Plummer M, et al. *Helicobacter pylori* multiplex serology and risk of noncardia and cardia gastric cancer: A case cohort study and meta-analysis. International Journal of Epidemiology. 2023;**52**(4):1197-1208. DOI: 10.1093/ije/dyad007

[67] Butt J, Varga MG, Wang T, Tsugane S, Shimazu T, Zheng W, et al. Smoking, *Helicobacter pylori* serology, and gastric cancer risk in prospective studies from China, Japan, and Korea. Cancer Prevention Research. 2019;**12**(10):667-674. DOI: 10.1158/1940-6207.CAPR-190238

[68] Cai H, Ye F, Michel A, Murphy G, Sasazuki S, Taylor PR, et al. *Helicobacter pylori* blood biomarker for gastric cancer risk in East Asia. International Journal of Epidemiology. 2016;**45**(3):774-781. DOI: 10.1093/ije/dyw078

[69] Pak K, Junga Z, Mertz A, Singla M. The patterns and associated cost of serologic testing for *Helicobacter pylori* in the U.S. military health system. Military Medicine. 2020;**185**(9-10):e1417-e1419. DOI: 10.1093/milmed/usaa141

[70] Godbole G, Mégraud F, Bessède E. Review: Diagnosis of *Helicobacter pylori* infection. Helicobacter. 2020;**25**(Suppl. 1):e12735. DOI: 10.1111/hel.12735

[71] Charitos IA, D'Agostino D, Topi S, Bottalico L. 40 years of *Helicobacter*

pylori: A revolution in biomedical thought. Gastroenterology Insights. 2021;**12**(2):111-135. DOI: 10.3390/gastroent12020011

[72] Dahlén G, Hassan H, Blomqvist S, Carlén A. Rapid urease test (RUT) for evaluation of urease activity in oral bacteria in vitro and in supragingival dental plaque ex vivo. BMC Oral Health. 2018;**18**(1):89. DOI: 10.1186/s12903-018-0541-3

[73] Vazirzadeh J, Moghim S, Falahi J, Narimani T, Rafiei R, Karbasizadeh V. Comparison of four invasive methods for diagnosis of *Helicobacter pylori* infection: Fluorescence in situ hybridization, histology, culture, rapid urease test. Molecular Genetics, Microbiology and Virology. 2020;**35**(2):123-128. DOI: 10.3103/s0891416820020111

[74] Young KA, Akyon Y, Rampton DS, Barton SGRG, Allaker RP, Hardie JM, et al. Quantitative culture of *Helicobacter pylori* from gastric juice: The potential for transmission. Journal of Medical Microbiology. 2000;**49**(4):343-347. DOI: 10.1099/0022-1317-49-4-343

[75] Gantuya B, El Serag HB, Saruuljavkhlan B, Azzaya D, Matsumoto T, Uchida T, et al. Advantage of 16S rRNA amplicon sequencing in *Helicobacter pylori* diagnosis. Helicobacter. 2021;**26**(3):e12790. DOI: 10.1111/hel.12790

[76] Frickmann H, Zautner AE, Moter A, Kikhney J, Hagen RM, Stender H, et al. Fluorescence in situ hybridization (FISH) in the microbiological diagnostic routine laboratory: A review. Critical Reviews in Microbiology. 2017;**43**(3):263-293. DOI: 10.3109/1040841X.2016.1169990

[77] Zhang Y, Gu H, Shi Z, Chen W, Li A, Ye W, et al. High prevalence of *Helicobacter pylori* mixed infections identified by multilocus sequence typing in Ningbo, China. Frontiers in Microbiology. 2023;**14**:1207878. DOI: 10.3389/fmicb.2023.1207878

[78] Kocsmár É, Kocsmár I, Buzás GM, Szirtes I, Wacha J, Takáts A, et al. *Helicobacter pylori* heteroresistance to clarithromycin in adults—New data by in situ detection and improved concept. Helicobacter. 2020;**25**(1):e12670. DOI: 10.1111/hel.12670

[79] Wongphutorn P, Chomvarin C, Sripa B, Namwat W, Faksri K. Detection and genotyping of *Helicobacter pylori* in saliva versus stool samples from asymptomatic individuals in Northeastern Thailand reveals intra-host tissue specific *H. pylori* subtypes. BMC Microbiology. 2018;**18**(1):10. DOI: 10.1186/s12866-018-1150-7

[80] Shiotani A, Roy P, Lu H, Graham DY. *Helicobacter pylori* diagnosis and therapy in the era of antimicrobial stewardship. Therapeutic Advances in Gastroenterology. 2021;**14**:17562848211064080

[81] Chey WD, Wong BC. American College of Gastroenterology guideline on the management of *Helicobacter pylori* infection. American Journal of Gastroenterology. 2007;**102**(8):1808-1825

[82] O'Connor A, Molina-Infante J, Gisbert JP, O'Morain C. Treatment of *Helicobacter pylori* infection 2013. Helicobacter. 2013;**18**(Suppl 1):58-65

[83] Sánchez-Delgado J, García-Iglesias P, Castro-Fernández M, Bory F, Barenys M, Bujanda L. High-dose, ten-day esomeprazole, amoxicillin and metronidazole triple therapy achieves high *Helicobacter pylori* eradication rates. Alimentary Pharmacology & Therapeutics. 2012;**36**(2):190-196

[84] Graham DY, Canaan Y, Maher J, Wiener G, Hulten KG, Kalfus IN. Rifabutin-based triple therapy (RHB-105) for *Helicobacter pylori* eradication: A double-blind, randomized, controlled trial. Annals of Internal Medicine. 2020;**172**(12):795-802

[85] Fallone CA. The current role of Vonoprazan in *Helicobacter pylori* treatment. Gastroenterology. 2022;**163**(3):572-574

[86] Zullo A, De Francesco V, Hassan C, Ridola L, Repici A, Bruzzese V, et al. Modified sequential therapy regimens for *Helicobacter pylori* eradication: A systematic review. Digestive and Liver Disease. 2013;**45**(1):18-22

[87] Molina-Infante J, Lucendo AJ, Angueira T, Rodriguez-Tellez M, Perez-Aisa A, Balboa A, et al. Optimised empiric triple and concomitant therapy for *Helicobacter pylori* eradication in clinical practice: The OPTRICON study. Alimentary Pharmacology & Therapeutics. 2015;**41**(6):581-589

[88] Hsu PI, Kao SS, Wu DC, Chen WC, Peng NJ, Yu HC, et al. A randomized controlled study comparing reverse hybrid therapy and standard triple therapy for *Helicobacter pylori* infection. Medicine (Baltimore). 2015;**94**(48):e2104

[89] Hsu PI, Tsay FW, Kao JY, Peng NJ, Tsai KW, Tsai TJ, et al. Equivalent efficacies of reverse hybrid and concomitant therapies in first-line treatment of *Helicobacter pylori* infection. Journal of Gastroenterology and Hepatology. 2020;**35**(10):1731-1737

[90] Kuo CH, Hsu PI, Kuo FC, Wang SS, Hu HM, Liu CJ. Comparison of 10-day bismuth quadruple therapy with high-dose metronidazole or levofloxacin for second-line *Helicobacter pylori* therapy: A randomized controlled trial. The Journal of Antimicrobial Chemotherapy. 2013;**68**(1):222-228

[91] Fu W, Song Z, Zhou L, Xue Y, Ding Y, Suo B, et al. Randomized clinical trial: Esomeprazole, bismuth, levofloxacin, and amoxicillin or cefuroxime as first-line eradication regimens for *Helicobacter pylori* infection. Digestive Diseases and Sciences. 2017;**62**(6):1580-1589

[92] Micromedex. Merative. Available from: www.micromedexsolutions.com [Accessed: March 14, 2025].

Chapter 2

Helicobacter pylori: Pathogenesis, Clinical Impact, and Modern Treatment Approaches

Arti Wongcha-Um, Tinpawee Thongkongthun, Ratha-korn Vilaichone and Varocha Mahachai

Abstract

Helicobacter pylori infection remains a global health concern, with rising antibiotic resistance compromising the efficacy of standard eradication therapies. This chapter introduces a novel approach: PCAPs-based therapy (Proton pump inhibitor, Clarithromycin, Amoxicillin, and Probiotics), which integrates antimicrobial, acid-suppressive, and microbiota-modulating strategies. We explore the epidemiology, pathogenic mechanisms, and clinical manifestations of *H. pylori* infection, with a focus on evolving resistance patterns. Emphasis is placed on the role of host-microbiome interactions, the rationale for probiotic adjuncts, and clinical evidence supporting PCAPs regimens. Through comprehensive review and expert commentary, this chapter advocates for a paradigm shift in the treatment of *H. pylori*, aligning with precision medicine principles to enhance eradication rates and reduce recurrence.

Keywords: *Helicobacter pylori* infection, *H. pylori* eradication therapy, *H. pylori* antibiotic resistance, PCAPs regimen for *H. pylori*, probiotics in *H. pylori* treatment

1. Introduction

Helicobacter pylori (*H. pylori*) is a helical, microaerophilic gram-negative bacterium that colonizes the human stomach and is one of the most prevalent chronic infections worldwide [1, 2]. First discovered in 1982 by Barry Marshall and Robin Warren, *H. pylori*'s role in gastritis and peptic ulcer disease has revolutionized gastroenterology [3]. In 2005, Marshall and Warren were awarded the Nobel Prize for their discovery that *H. pylori* causes chronic active gastritis and peptic ulcers, transforming these conditions from chronic, often intractable illnesses into infections that can be cured with targeted antibiotics and acid suppression [3]. *H. pylori* is now formally recognized as an infectious disease (included in the ICD-11 classification), and eradication of this pathogen is considered a key strategy for preventing its associated gastrointestinal diseases [1, 4].

H. pylori is a spiral-shaped bacilli (~3 μm long) with multiple unipolar flagella that confer motility and an ability to penetrate the gastric mucus layer. The bacterium produces high levels of urease, enabling it to locally neutralize gastric acid and survive in the harsh acidic environment of the stomach. This unique adaptation allows *H. pylori* to establish lifelong colonization in the human gastric mucosa. *H. pylori* infection induces a chronic gastric mucosal inflammation (chronic active gastritis) in all infected hosts [1]. While the majority of infections remain asymptomatic or cause only mild dyspepsia, a significant minority of individuals develop severe gastroduodenal pathologies over time [1, 2]. Notably, *H. pylori* is the etiologic agent in most peptic ulcer disease and is strongly linked to gastric malignancies, including gastric adenocarcinoma and gastric mucosa-associated lymphoid tissue (MALT) lymphoma [1]. In 1994, the World Health Organization's International Agency for Research on Cancer classified *H. pylori* as a Group 1 carcinogen due to its causal relationship with gastric cancer. Globally, *H. pylori* infection is identified in the vast majority of non-cardia gastric cancers and is considered the dominant risk factor for this cancer, which remains one of the leading causes of cancer mortality worldwide [2].

H. pylori infection carries tremendous global public health significance. It is estimated that approximately half of the world's population harbors this bacterium [1]. A 2017 meta-analysis extrapolated that around 4.4 billion individuals were infected with *H. pylori* in 2015 [5]. The prevalence of infection varies markedly by region and socioeconomic status: for example, *H. pylori* is nearly universal in some low-income countries, with pooled prevalence ~70% or higher in regions of Africa and parts of Asia, while more developed regions like Western Europe and North America report adult prevalence around 30% [5, 6]. Among individual countries surveyed, prevalence ranges from under 20% (e.g., ~19% in Switzerland) to over 85% (e.g., ~88% in Nigeria) [5]. Such geographic variation reflects differences in living conditions, sanitation, and birth cohort effects. In general, infection is acquired primarily in childhood and is associated with overcrowding, poor hygiene, and lower socioeconomic status during early life [6]. Countries undergoing socioeconomic development have witnessed a birth-cohort effect, with significantly lower *H. pylori* prevalence in younger generations compared to older ones, portending a natural decline in overall prevalence in coming decades [6]. Despite this decline in some regions, *H. pylori* remains one of the most common human pathogens. Because of its ubiquity and its role in serious diseases, there is intense ongoing research into improved treatment strategies and preventive measures including vaccine development to reduce the global burden of *H. pylori* infection.

This chapter provides a comprehensive review of *H. pylori*, focusing on its causes and transmission, the spectrum of clinical symptoms and disease associations, and current as well as emerging treatment options. We discuss how host and bacterial factors influence disease outcomes, summarize the clinical manifestations ranging from asymptomatic gastritis to peptic ulcer disease and gastric cancer, and detail the recommended therapeutic regimens for *H. pylori* eradication. Recent advances—such as novel acid suppressants (potassium-competitive acid blockers) and vaccine research—are highlighted in the context of challenges like rising antibiotic resistance. By emulating a peer-reviewed scientific discourse with up-to-date evidence, this chapter aims to serve as an authoritative resource on *H. pylori* for clinicians and researchers alike.

DOI: http://dx.doi.org/10.5772/intechopen.1011730

2. Causes

2.1 Transmission and epidemiological risk factors

H. pylori is typically acquired via person-to-person transmission, most often in childhood. The exact modes of transmission are not completely characterized, but multiple routes have been implicated. Fecal-oral transmission is supported by the detection of *H. pylori* DNA in feces and the association of infection with poor sanitation and contaminated water supplies. Oral-oral transmission is also considered important, given that *H. pylori* can be isolated from saliva and dental plaque; intrafamilial clustering of infection is well-documented, suggesting that close contact (e.g., between parents and children or among siblings) facilitates spread. A gastric-oral route from vomitus has been proposed as well: episodes of gastroenteritis in an infected individual (especially with vomiting) can expel *H. pylori* from the stomach and expose close contacts. Notably, a prospective study in households showed that exposure to an *H. pylori*-infected family member with vomiting significantly increased the risk of new *H. pylori* infection in contacts (odds ratio ~ 6), implicating vomitus as a highly infectious vehicle. These lines of evidence indicate that *H. pylori* spreads primarily via direct human-to-human pathways (fecal/oral, oral/oral, or gastric/oral), rather than through an environmental reservoir. Iatrogenic transmission via inadequately disinfected endoscopes has also been reported in rare cases, but this is exceptional.

The infection is usually acquired in early childhood and tends to persist life-long unless treated. In developing countries, the majority of children become infected before age 10, whereas in developed countries, acquisition is less common in childhood and more often delayed or altogether avoided. Once established, *H. pylori* infection generally remains chronic, with very low spontaneous clearance rates. Reinfection after successful eradication is uncommon in adults in developed regions (typically <3% per year) but can be higher in high-prevalence settings (up to 10% or more per year).

A number of epidemiological risk factors for acquiring *H. pylori* have been identified, most of which are surrogates for exposure to the above transmission routes. Socioeconomic status and living conditions in childhood are paramount: lower socioeconomic conditions, overcrowded households, limited access to clean water, and poor sanitation all markedly increase the risk of *H. pylori* infection [6]. Children living in densely populated homes or attending daycare with poor hygiene may be more likely to become infected. Geography reflects these disparities—infection prevalence is the highest in regions such as Africa, South Asia, and parts of Latin America where many communities have limited sanitation, whereas prevalence is much lower in North America, Northern Europe, and Australia [5, 6]. Within countries, underprivileged and indigenous populations often show higher infection rates; for example, *H. pylori* is more common in immigrant populations originating from high-prevalence countries [6]. Age is also a factor: older age groups have higher *H. pylori* prevalence than younger age groups in the same region, largely due to higher infection rates in past decades and birth-cohort differences [6]. Household transmission plays a key role—having an infected parent or sibling greatly increases a child's risk of infection, explaining familial clustering of *H. pylori*.

Certain behavioral factors can influence *H. pylori* transmission or persistence. Poor food hygiene and consumption of contaminated water or improperly washed vegetables could allow fecal-oral spread. Overcrowding facilitates oral-oral transmission among family members. In contrast, breastfeeding in infancy may offer some protection by transfer of maternal antibodies. There is also evidence that smoking and tobacco exposure are associated with a higher likelihood of *H. pylori* infection and may impair clearance. Studies indicate smokers have a significantly higher risk of being *H. pylori*-positive than non-smokers (one analysis found a risk ratio ~5 for infection in smokers) [7, 8]. Additionally, smokers are nearly twice as likely to experience treatment failure when undergoing *H. pylori* eradication therapy (meta-analysis OR ~1.95 for eradication failure in smokers) [9]. The mechanisms may include smoking-induced changes in gastric physiology or immune response that favors persistence of the bacterium.

In summary, *H. pylori* infection is usually acquired via interpersonal transmission in early life under conditions of close contact and suboptimal hygiene. Key risk factors include low socioeconomic status, crowding, and having infected family members, which together explain the high prevalence of *H. pylori* in developing regions and socioeconomically disadvantaged groups. Public health improvements in sanitation and living conditions are believed to underlie the declining *H. pylori* prevalence observed in many industrialized countries over recent decades [6].

3. Host and bacterial factors influencing disease susceptibility

While *H. pylori* infection is common, the clinical outcomes vary widely—ranging from asymptomatic carriage to severe ulcer disease or gastric malignancy. This variability is determined by a complex interplay of host factors, bacterial virulence, and environmental influences. Only a subset of infected persons ever develop serious disease, and understanding the modulating factors is key to identifying those at risk.

Host genetic factors have been shown to influence the host inflammatory responses to *H. pylori* and subsequent tissue damage. For example, polymorphisms in pro-inflammatory cytokine genes can affect the intensity of gastritis. Notably, certain interleukin-1 beta (IL-1β) gene polymorphisms that result in higher IL-1β production are associated with an increased risk of gastric atrophy and cancer in *H. pylori*-infected individuals [10]. IL-1β is a potent acid inhibitor; genetically high IL-1β responders may develop hypochlorhydria and multifocal atrophic gastritis when infected, which promotes carcinogenesis. Similarly, polymorphisms in the tumor necrosis factor-alpha (TNF-α) gene and others have been linked to differential risks of gastric cancer. Host blood group has also been implicated: individuals with blood type O were historically noted to have higher prevalence of duodenal ulcers in *H. pylori* infection, possibly due to *H. pylori*'s preference for binding to Lewis b antigens highly expressed in type O secretors. Moreover, host immune response genes (e.g., certain HLA alleles) may affect susceptibility to *H. pylori* or propensity for more severe inflammation. Physiological factors like gastric acid secretion levels can modulate disease expression—hosts with high acid output tend to develop antral-predominant gastritis and duodenal ulcers, whereas those who mount pangastritis with acid loss are more prone to gastric ulcer and cancer. Lifestyle factors such as diet and co-morbid conditions also play a role; for instance, high dietary salt intake has been shown to exacerbate *H. pylori*-induced gastric injury in animal models, and smoking or NSAID use synergistically increases risk of ulcer complications in infected persons.

On the microbial side, *H. pylori* strain heterogeneity is a critical determinant of pathogenicity. Clinical outcomes correlate strongly with the presence of specific

DOI: http://dx.doi.org/10.5772/intechopen.1011730

bacterial virulence factors. The best-characterized is the Cag pathogenicity island, a 40-kb genomic island present in ~50–70% of Western *H. pylori* strains (and virtually all East Asian strains). This island encodes a type IV secretion system that injects the CagA protein into gastric epithelial cells. CagA (cytotoxin-associated gene A) is a major virulence factor that dysregulates host cell signaling: it triggers pro-inflammatory pathways (e.g., NF-κB), perturbs cell polarity and adhesion, and can stimulate cell proliferation. Infections with CagA-positive *H. pylori* strains lead to more intense neutrophilic inflammation and tissue damage than CagA-negative strains. Epidemiologically, CagA+ strains are associated with a greater risk of peptic ulcer (odds of ulcer disease are higher) and a significantly increased risk of gastric cancer. In fact, colonization by a CagA-positive strain confers additional oncogenic risk beyond *H. pylori* infection alone; CagA is often termed a bacterial oncoprotein for its role in promoting gastric tumorigenesis [2]. East Asian CagA variants may be especially potent, which may partly explain the higher gastric cancer rates in regions like Japan and Korea where virtually all *H. pylori* carry CagA. Another key virulence factor is VacA (vacuolating cytotoxin A), a secreted toxin present in all *H. pylori* strains but with different allelic types. VacA causes cell vacuolation and mitochondrial damage. Certain VacA genotypes (s1/m1 alleles) produce more active toxin and are linked to greater tissue injury and disease severity, whereas s2/m2 strains are less virulent. Strains that are CagA- positive typically also have the more cytotoxic VacA alleles, creating a synergistically virulent profile. Other *H. pylori* factors contribute as well: BabA (blood-group antigen binding adhesin) allows the bacterium to adhere to Lewis b blood group antigens on gastric epithelial cells, facilitating colonization; OipA (outer inflammatory protein) is associated with enhanced inflammation; and DupA (duodenal ulcer promoting gene) has been linked by some studies to duodenal ulcer risk. The plasticity region of the *H. pylori* genome and various secretion system effectors further modulate interactions with the host. In summary, bacterial strains that harbor a complement of high-virulence determinants (CagA positivity, toxigenic VacA, adherence factors) incite greater inflammation and epithelial damage, predisposing the host to ulcers and gastric neoplasia, whereas less virulent strains often lead to mild gastritis or asymptomatic infection [2].

Infected individuals' outcomes thus depend on this triad: the host genetic makeup and immune inflammatory response capacity, the virulence of the particular *H. pylori* strain, and environmental factors (diet, smoking, co-infections, etc.). For example, a person with pro-inflammatory cytokine polymorphisms infected by a CagA+/VacA s1m1 strain, who smokes and has a high-salt diet, would be at substantially elevated risk for severe gastritis and gastric cancer. In contrast, a host with a blunted inflammatory genotype infected by a less virulent strain might remain asymptomatic. This variability underscores why only a fraction of the ~50% of humans infected go on to develop overt disease. It also suggests that targeted interventions (such as eradicating particularly high-risk infections or modifying co-factors like smoking and diet) could mitigate disease burden.

4. Symptoms and clinical manifestations

H. pylori infection induces chronic gastritis in virtually all colonized individuals, but the clinical presentation ranges from a complete lack of symptoms to life-threatening complications. Approximately 80% of *H. pylori*-infected individuals are asymptomatic and unaware of their infection [1]. *H. pylori* causes an ongoing but subclinical inflammation of the gastric mucosa that may only be detectable by biopsy (histologic gastritis) without overt clinical signs. Even asymptomatic infection can lead to insidious mucosal damage over decades, potentially progressing to atrophic gastritis or other sequelae in some cases. However, many people coexist with the organism lifelong and never develop significant clinical illness.

When symptoms do occur, they are usually related to gastroduodenal mucosal damage caused by *H. pylori*'s inflammatory effects. The most common manifestation is dyspepsia, a syndrome of upper abdominal discomfort or pain, bloating, early satiety, and nausea. *H. pylori* is a major cause of chronic gastritis and has been linked to functional dyspepsia in some patients [1]. In many cases *H. pylori*-associated dyspepsia is mild, but it can be persistent. Notably, randomized trials have shown that a subset of patients with non-ulcer dyspepsia experience significant symptom improvement after *H. pylori* eradication, implying that the infection was contributing to their dyspeptic symptoms. Thus, current guidelines often recommend a "test-and-treat" approach for *H. pylori* in younger patients with uninvestigated dyspepsia, given the possibility that treating the infection will alleviate symptoms.

More pronounced clinical syndromes arise when *H. pylori* causes peptic ulcer disease (PUD). *H. pylori* is etiologically involved in the majority of peptic ulcers: approximately 90% of duodenal ulcers and 70–80% of gastric ulcers are attributable to *H. pylori* infection, with most of the remainder linked to NSAID use [1]. Ulcers result from the interplay of bacterial-induced mucosal damage and alterations in gastric acid secretion. Antral-predominant *H. pylori* gastritis increases gastrin release and acid production, which in turn contributes to duodenal ulcer formation; in the stomach, *H. pylori*-related mucosal inflammation impairs defenses and promotes ulceration especially in the presence of risk factors like NSAIDs. Clinically, peptic ulcers due to *H. pylori* typically cause recurrent epigastric pain that may be burning or gnawing, often occurring when the stomach is empty; classically, duodenal ulcer pain is relieved by food, whereas gastric ulcer pain can be exacerbated by eating. Other dyspeptic symptoms such as bloating, heartburn, or nausea can accompany. A significant proportion of ulcer patients have only mild symptoms or even none at all, until complications arise. Ulcer complications include bleeding presenting as melena or hematemesis, obstruction, and perforation, all of which are medical emergencies. *H. pylori*-associated ulcers are prone to bleeding if untreated, and indeed *H. pylori* is a leading cause of non-variceal upper gastrointestinal hemorrhage globally. When *H. pylori* infection is cured, ulcer recurrence rates drop dramatically, reaffirming the causative role of the bacterium. Thus, identification and eradication of *H. pylori* is standard of care in all patients with confirmed peptic ulcer disease.

Beyond peptic ulcers, *H. pylori* is implicated in a spectrum of other gastric pathologies. One notable entity is gastric MALT lymphoma (mucosa-associated lymphoid tissue lymphoma), a low-grade B-cell lymphoma of the stomach. Chronic *H. pylori* infection drives lymphoid proliferation in the gastric mucosa, and in about 1% of infected persons, this can lead to clonal expansion of B-cells and lymphoma development. Over 90% of gastric MALT lymphomas are associated with *H. pylori* infection. The clinical signs may be nonspecific (dyspepsia, mild pain) or absent; it is often discovered on endoscopy as an abnormal mucosal lesion. Importantly, early-stage *H. pylori*-associated MALT lymphoma can regress completely with antibiotic eradication of *H. pylori* in ~75% of cases, representing a remarkable example of oncogenesis reversal by treating an infection. The recognition of this association has made *H. pylori* eradication the first-line therapy for localized gastric MALT lymphoma, often obviating the need for chemotherapy or radiation if the lymphoma regresses.

The most ominous outcome of *H. pylori* infection is the development of gastric adenocarcinoma. Chronic *H. pylori* gastritis is the single strongest risk factor for non-cardia gastric cancer. The pathogenesis follows the well-described Correa cascade: long-standing *H. pylori* infection causes chronic active gastritis, which in some individuals progresses to multifocal atrophic gastritis with loss of gastric glands and intestinal metaplasia of the stomach lining; these pre-malignant changes can further progress to dysplasia and eventually carcinoma over decades. This sequence is influenced by host and bacterial factors as discussed.

H. pylori is estimated to account for roughly 89% of all distal (non-cardia) gastric cancers worldwide [2]. Prospective studies have shown that *H. pylori*-infected persons have a significantly elevated risk, six-fold or more, of developing gastric cancer compared to uninfected counterparts, particularly if infected with high-risk strains. Gastric cancer arising in the context of *H. pylori* typically presents late, with symptoms like weight loss, persistent abdominal pain, anorexia, or early satiety; often it is detected only after the tumor causes gastric outlet obstruction, bleeding, or perforation. Given the poor prognosis of advanced gastric cancer, there is intense interest in preventing cancer by eradicating *H. pylori* at the pre-malignant stage. There is evidence that *H. pylori* eradication can partially reverse or halt the progression of atrophic gastritis and thereby reduce gastric cancer risk, especially if done before irreversible dysplasia has developed. Several population-based interventions (e.g., in high-incidence regions like Japan and China) are exploring screen-and-treat programs for *H. pylori* as a gastric cancer prevention strategy. For instance, Japan now recommends *H. pylori* testing and treatment in all diagnosed gastritis patients as an effort to reduce future cancer incidence.

In addition to these well-established gastric diseases, *H. pylori* infection has been associated with various extra-gastric manifestations. Though causal links are less clear, epidemiologic studies suggest *H. pylori* may contribute to unexplained iron-deficiency anemia and idiopathic thrombocytopenic purpura (ITP) through autoimmune mechanisms [2]. In many patients with refractory iron-deficiency or ITP, treating *H. pylori* can lead to improvement in anemia or platelet counts, respectively, supporting a contributory role. Other suggested associations include cardiovascular disease, neurological disorders (e.g., Parkinson's disease), and metabolic syndrome, but these remain controversial and are not proven causal. The most accepted extra-gastric links are with iron deficiency and ITP, for which some guidelines advise testing for and eradicating *H. pylori* as part of management.

To summarize, the clinical spectrum of *H. pylori* infection ranges from silent gastritis to severe ulcer disease and gastric neoplasia. Many infected individuals remain asymptomatic, but all have some degree of gastric mucosal inflammation, which can progress insidiously. Symptomatic infection commonly manifests as dyspepsia or peptic ulcer disease, with *H. pylori* being a principal cause of both chronic gastritis symptoms and ulcer complications like bleeding. *H. pylori* is unique among bacterial pathogens in its carcinogenic potential, being the instigator of most gastric cancers and MALT lymphomas. The variability in outcome is governed by the factors outlined earlier. From a clinical perspective, this means that all *H. pylori*-infected patients are at least at some elevated risk and can potentially benefit from eradication therapy, even if asymptomatic, to prevent future complications [1]. Indeed, leading experts now consider *H. pylori* gastritis an infectious disease that merits treatment in essentially all who test positive [4]. The decision to test for *H. pylori* is often driven by clinical context (ulcer history, dyspepsia, family history of gastric cancer, etc.), but once an infection is confirmed, current recommendation advocates eradication therapy to forestall the possible serious outcomes.

5. Treatment options

The goal of *H. pylori* treatment is successful eradication, thereby allowing gastritis to resolve and preventing recurrence of ulcers or development of cancer. Achieving a durable cure for *H. pylori* is feasible but can be challenging due to the bacterium's ability to reside in the protective mucus niche and the growing problem of antibiotic resistance. This section will detail the current standard pharmacological therapies, discuss antibiotic resistance and the role of susceptibility testing (including novel molecular diagnostics), and review non-pharmacological adjuncts and preventive strategies. Recent advances on a new acid-suppressing agent Potassium-competitive acid blocker (PCAB), in eradication therapy and vaccine development will be on descend.

6. Pharmacological eradication therapies

Combination antibiotic therapy with an acid-suppressant is the cornerstone of *H. pylori* treatment. Monotherapy is ineffective due to *H. pylori*'s ability to rapidly develop resistance; instead, regimens combining two or more antibiotics with a proton-pump inhibitor (PPI) have been used to achieve synergistic eradication and high cure rates. The PPI (or other acid suppressor) is a critical component because raising intragastric pH improves antibiotic stability and penetration to the bacteria. Bismuth compounds, which have direct bactericidal and mucosal protective effects, are included in certain regimens as well. Treatment is given for a finite course (typically 10–14 days). Successful eradication is defined by post-treatment testing (urea breath test, stool antigen, or biopsy) confirming the absence of *H. pylori*.

Over the past two decades, a number of first-line regimens have been developed and refined. The optimal choice of regimen depends on factors such as local antibiotic resistance patterns, patient antibiotic tolerances/allergies, and prior exposure. The major recommended first-line therapies include:

- PPI triple therapy (clarithromycin triple therapy): This classic regimen consists of a PPI + clarithromycin + a second antibiotic, usually amoxicillin, or metronidazole in penicillin-allergic patients, given twice daily for 14 days. Standard triple therapy was for many years the empirical treatment of choice and in the 1990s achieved eradication rates of ~85–90% in clinical trials when *H. pylori* strains were susceptible [11]. However, its efficacy has declined substantially in most regions due to rising clarithromycin resistance. Clarithromycin resistance in *H. pylori* is mediated by 23S rRNA point mutations and leads to treatment failure in the majority of cases. Meta-analyses have shown that if the infecting strain is clarithromycin-resistant, the success rate of clarithromycin-based triple therapy declines by about 55 percentage points compared to susceptible strains [11]. For example, cure rates were ~90% in clarithromycin-sensitive infections but <35–40% when the strain was resistant [11]. Unfortunately, the prevalence of clarithromycin- resistant *H. pylori* now exceeds 15–20% in many parts of the world and >30% in some areas, rendering triple therapy inadequate in a large fraction of patients. Likewise, metronidazole resistance can reduce triple therapy efficacy, though high-dose or longer therapy can partly overcome it. Due to these trends, most guidelines now recommend clarithromycin-based triple therapy only in regions or patient groups where *H. pylori* clarithromycin resistance is known to be low (<15%). When used, 14-day duration is advised (7-day regimens are inferior). In settings with higher resistance or unknown patterns, other regimens have replaced triple therapy.

- Bismuth quadruple therapy: A highly effective, resistance-resilient regimen consisting of a PPI + bismuth + tetracycline + a nitroimidazole (usually metronidazole), given for 10–14 days. Bismuth quadruple therapy (BQT) has become a mainstay first-line treatment, if available, especially in areas with high dual resistance to clarithromycin and metronidazole. The addition of bismuth and tetracycline provides potent bactericidal activity that is largely unaffected by clarithromycin resistance. Typical eradication rates for 14-day bismuth quadruple therapy are in the 80–90% range in intention-to-treat analyses [12]. Even when metronidazole resistance is present, the synergy of multiple drugs in BQT often still yields acceptable cure rates (metronidazole resistance can be partially overcome by the bismuth and high-dose tetracycline). This regimen's drawbacks include a relatively high pill burden and potential side effects (e.g., bismuth can cause dark stools/tongue, tetracycline can cause photosensitivity, metronidazole can cause nausea and a metallic taste, and alcohol must be avoided with metronidazole). Nonetheless, BQT is recommended as a first-line option in European (Maastricht VI) and North American guidelines, particularly where clarithromycin resistance is common. It is also the regimen of choice for patients with prior macrolide exposure or a penicillin allergy. A 10-day course can be used, but a 14-day course is associated with slightly higher efficacy. Real-world studies show BQT achieving around 80%+ cure rates in many populations, outperforming triple therapy in resistant infections [12].

- Non-bismuth quadruple concomitant therapy: So-called "concomitant" therapy includes a PPI and three antibiotics given concurrently (usually clarithromycin, amoxicillin, and metronidazole or tinidazole) for 10–14 days. Concomitant therapy leverages four drugs to raise eradication rates and has shown high efficacy (~90% in clinical trials) because it is likely to contain at least two active antibiotics even if resistance is present to one. For instance, if clarithromycin resistance exists, amoxicillin + nitroimidazole can still work, and vice versa. Concomitant therapy for 14 days is recommended by many experts as an alternative first-line regimen in regions with high dual resistance. A variant is hybrid therapy, which starts as PPI + amoxicillin for 7 days, then in the second week adds clarithromycin + nitroimidazole (effectively sequential addition, but with amoxicillin continued throughout the 14 days). However, concomitant (all four drugs together from the start) has largely superseded sequential/hybrid strategies because of its simplicity and excellent efficacy. The main limitation is increased risk of side effects due to multiple antibiotics; still, studies indicate patients generally tolerate concomitant therapy reasonably, and compliance is crucial for success.

- Sequential therapy: An older strategy where one set of antibiotics is given in the first phase and another set in the second phase. For example, a 10-day sequential regimen might be: days 1–5 with PPI + amoxicillin, then days 6–10 with PPI + clarithromycin + metronidazole. The rationale was to use amoxicillin first to reduce bacterial load and potentially break resistance, then follow with the other two antibiotics. While sequential therapy demonstrated high eradication rates (~85–90%) in some trials, subsequent studies and meta-analyses yielded mixed results, and its complexity can confuse patients. In practice, concomitant therapy (which is like sequential but with overlap) has similar or better efficacy and is easier to comply. Thus, sequential therapy is now less commonly recommended, except perhaps in certain cases of clarithromycin resistance where initial amoxicillin "pretreatment" might boost effectiveness.

- Levofloxacin-containing regimens: Fluoroquinolone-based therapies are often used as second-line or rescue treatments after failure of first-line therapy, but they can also be first-line options in areas with low quinolone resistance. A typical levofloxacin triple regimen is PPI + levofloxacin + amoxicillin for 10–14 days. When fluoroquinolone resistance rates are low (<10%), this regimen can achieve ~80–90% eradication. However, levofloxacin resistance in *H. pylori* (due to gyrA mutations) has been increasing, and resistance significantly lowers success. In a patient who has failed clarithromycin-based therapy, a levofloxacin regimen is a common next choice (unless the patient was previously exposed to quinolones for other reasons). Additionally, levofloxacin quadruple (PPI + bismuth + levofloxacin + tetracycline or amoxicillin) and fluoroquinolone sequential therapies have been studied. European guidelines suggest that after the first failure on clarithromycin triple, a bismuth quadruple or levofloxacin triple can be used as second-line, depending on availability and local patterns.

- High-dose dual therapy: An emerging approach revisiting an old concept—using just a PPI and amoxicillin, but at high and frequent dosing, to eradicate *H. pylori*. Amoxicillin resistance in *H. pylori* is extremely rare, and amoxicillin's effectiveness is time-dependent (better at prolonged high concentrations). By using a high-dose PPI to maintain near-maximum acid suppression together with high-dose amoxicillin given 3–4 times daily, intragastric antibiotic levels are sustained, and the bacteria are continuously suppressed during growth. Recent studies, especially from Asia, have shown that 14-day high-dose PPI + amoxicillin dual therapy can achieve eradication rates around 85–90%, comparable to standard triple or quadruple regimens [13, 14]. For example, one trial of high-dose rabeprazole (20 mg QID) plus amoxicillin 750 mg QID reported ~90% cure as first-line therapy [13]. This strategy's advantages are the use of only one antibiotic-minimizing side effects and avoidance of clarithromycin or metronidazole in populations with high resistance. However, it requires impeccable patient compliance due to the very frequent dosing, and its success likely hinges on using a very potent acid inhibitor. The advent of potassium-competitive acid blockers has renewed interest in dual therapy, because their stronger acid suppression may further enhance amoxicillin's effect. Some recent trials combining vonoprazan (a novel acid blocker) with amoxicillin have demonstrated encouraging eradication rates (~85–90%) with dual therapy [15].

- Rifabutin triple therapy, typically combining a proton pump inhibitor (PPI), amoxicillin, and rifabutin, is an effective option for *H. pylori* eradication. Rifabutin, an antibiotic mainly used for tuberculosis, is rarely subject to resistance in *H. pylori*, making it valuable in refractory infection. A generic regimen of PPI + amoxicillin + rifabutin (e.g., rifabutin 150 mg twice daily for 10–14 days) has historically been used as salvage therapy, with reported eradication rates of ~60–80% in multi-drug resistant cases. In the United States, the FDA has approved TALICIA®, a fixed-dose combination capsule (omeprazole 10 mg / amoxicillin 250 mg / rifabutin 12.5 mg) for *H. pylori* infection in adults, with an approved dosage of four capsules three times daily (TID) for 14 days (total daily dose: rifabutin 150 mg, amoxicillin 3000 mg, omeprazole 120 mg). This approval is not restricted to any particular line of therapy. Phase 3 trials in treatment-naïve patients demonstrated high efficacy, with ~84% eradication in the intent-to-treat (ITT) population and ~90% in adherent populations. The latest ACG Clinical Guideline (2024) includes rifabutin-based triple therapy as an alternative first-line empiric option when antibiotic susceptibility is unknown. Importantly, generic rifabutin triple regimens are not therapeutically equivalent to the fixed-dose TALICIA® formulation and should not be substituted. A potential but rare serious adverse effect of rifabutin is bone marrow suppression, so treatment courses are generally limited and require monitoring.

Other regimens and variations exist, for example, adding bismuth to levofloxacin triple to make a fluoroquinolone quadruple, or using furazolidone-based therapy in regions like China and Iran, or using doxycycline instead of tetracycline in quadruple therapy. The choices often depend on local availability of drugs and resistance patterns. **Table 1** provides an overview of several common first-line *H. pylori* treatment regimens and their typical eradication rates observed:

In clinical practice, current guideline recommendations (e.g., Maastricht VI Consensus [4], ACG 2017, Toronto Consensus) generally advise choosing a regimen that is likely to achieve ≥90% eradication in the local context. For many regions, this means avoiding clarithromycin triple therapy empirically and instead using either bismuth quadruple or a concomitant/non-bismuth quadruple as first-line. For

Regimen (duration)	Composition (daily doses)	Typical eradication rate (ITT)
Clarithromycin triple (14 days)	PPI + amoxicillin + clarithromycin (or metronidazole)	~70–85% (highly variable; <60% if CLA-resistant)
Bismuth quadruple (10–14 days)	PPI + bismuth + tetracycline + metronidazole	~80–90% in most populations
Concomitant quadruple (10–14 days)	PPI + clarithromycin + amoxicillin + metronidazole	~85–95% (robust even with single-drug resistance)
Levofloxacin triple (10–14 days)	PPI + levofloxacin + amoxicillin	~80–90% (when levofloxacin susceptibility is high)
High-dose dual (14 days)	High-dose PPI (e.g., bid or qid) + amoxicillin (q8h–6h)	~80–90% (with potent acid suppression)
Rifabutin triple (10–14 days)	Generic rifabutin triple (10–14 days; salvage use, ~60–80% efficacy)	~70–80% (salvage therapy after failures)
Rifabutin triple: TALICIA® (14 days)	Omeprazole 120 mg + amoxicillin 3000 mg + rifabutin 150 mg (fixed-dose capsule: 4 capsules TID with food)	~84% ITT, ~90% per-protocol in trials
P-CAB dual therapy	P-CAB + amoxicillin (high dose)	~90%
P-CAB triple therapy	P-CAB + amoxicillin + clarithromycin	~90%
P-CAB quadruple therapy	P-CAB + amoxicillin + clarithromycin + bismuth	>90%

Table 1.
Common H. pylori *eradication regimens and approximate efficacy.*

instance, the 2022 Maastricht VI report recommends routine susceptibility testing or, if not available, empirical use of bismuth quadruple or concomitant therapy in areas of known high resistance. In regions with low resistance where triple therapy is still used, it is critical to use the 14-day course and confirm eradication afterwards. After a first-line failure, second-line therapy should use antibiotics not previously used (to avoid resistance). A common strategy is: if clarithromycin-based therapy fails, use a bismuth quadruple or levofloxacin regimen next; if initial therapy was BQT, a switch to levofloxacin triple or a clarithromycin-containing regimen can be attempted. Salvage therapy after two failures often involves rifabutin triple or a furazolidone-based quadruple, depending on availability. Bismuth quadruple therapy and PCAB-based triple or quadruple also are highly effective and recommended in previous eradication failure. These stepwise approaches underscore the importance of having multiple lines of therapy due to growing resistance.

7. Antibiotic resistance and the role of susceptibility testing

Antibiotic resistance in *H. pylori* is the primary threat to effective treatment. As discussed, resistance to key antibiotics—especially clarithromycin, metronidazole, and levofloxacin—has escalated worldwide, undermining the success of standard regimens. For example, global clarithromycin resistance rates in *H. pylori* were reported at 15–20% on average by the 2010s, with higher resistance area (≥30%) in parts of Asia and Southern Europe [6, 16]. Metronidazole resistance is even more common (often 20–40% or higher), though its impact can sometimes be partially overcome by higher doses or combination therapy. Levofloxacin resistance has also risen with increased quinolone use in general practice. Amoxicillin and tetracycline resistance remain low (<5% generally), and thus these agents are reliable backbone drugs—this is why they often appear in rescue regimens.

The presence of resistance dramatically lowers eradication rates: a resistant subpopulation of *H. pylori* can survive the antibiotic course and lead to persistence of infection. After a treatment failure, the strain is often now resistant to one (or more) of the drugs used, making retreatment more difficult. Indeed, one study found that among patients who failed at least one therapy course, 86% of isolates were dual-resistant to clarithromycin and metronidazole [11]. Multidrug-resistant *H. pylori* (e.g., resistant to clarithromycin, metronidazole, and levofloxacin concurrently) are increasingly encountered in refractory cases. This trend necessitates either using bismuth quadruple regimens where resistance is less relevant or tailoring antibiotics based on susceptibility data when possible.

To address this, there is a strong push toward *H. pylori* culture and susceptibility testing or molecular resistance testing in the management of infection, particularly after a treatment failure. Traditional culture of *H. pylori* from gastric biopsies allows phenotypic sensitivity testing for antibiotics (agar dilution or E-test). However, culture is technically demanding—*H. pylori* is fastidious and grows slowly—and not widely available in routine practice in many regions. It can take up to 2 weeks to get results, and many developing countries lack laboratories for *H. pylori* culture. As an alternative, molecular diagnostics have emerged to detect resistance gene mutations directly from gastric biopsy DNA or stool samples. The prime example is PCR assays for clarithromycin resistance: these tests amplify portions of the 23S rRNA gene to identify the specific point mutations (A2142G, A2143G, etc.) that confer macrolide resistance [11]. Such PCR tests can return results rapidly and guide the choice of therapy and antibiotic stewardship for a proper selection of antibiotics. There are also molecular assays for mutations in gyrA (conferring fluoroquinolone resistance) and rdxA/frxA (metronidazole resistance markers), although the latter are less straightforward to interpret. Commercial kits, for example, gastric biopsy PCR kits and even a stool PCR test for *H. pylori* and clarithromycin resistance are now available and have been incorporated into practice in some areas. Molecular susceptibility testing is highlighted in recent consensus guidelines as a valuable tool: Maastricht VI, for example, emphasizes the use of novel molecular methods to inform therapy selection and improve outcomes [4]. The paradigm is shifting toward an individualized approach—"test for resistance and treat"—instead of empirical one-regimen-fits-all, at least in regions where resources allow.

In summary, rising antibiotic resistance in *H. pylori* has made antimicrobial stewardship and tailored therapy increasingly important. When available, susceptibility-guided therapy is ideal: one can choose an antibiotic combination to which the patient's strain is known to be susceptible, greatly increasing the chance of eradication. For example, if testing shows clarithromycin sensitivity, a clarithromycin regimen might be used; if not, a bismuth or levofloxacin regimen can be selected—this avoids giving the patient ineffective drugs and promotes antibiotic stewardship. Routine susceptibility testing before first-line treatment is not yet common except in research settings or areas of very high resistance because of cost and availability, but after multiple therapy failures, it is definitely recommended to perform culture or molecular testing to direct the next regimen. This approach will become more prevalent as molecular testing becomes faster and cheaper. Another implication of resistance is the push for new drugs or combinations in *H. pylori* therapy, as the traditional regimens lose efficacy. This includes the introduction of novel acid suppressants to maximize antibiotic effect and the exploration of non-antibiotic therapies. Ultimately, addressing *H. pylori* antibiotic resistance is crucial for maintaining high cure rates—either through better diagnostics to optimize therapy or through developing regimens that are less affected by resistance such as quadruple therapies or entirely new drug classes.

8. Recent advances: Novel acid suppression and therapeutics

One of the most significant recent pharmacological advances in *H. pylori* treatment is the development of potassium-competitive acid blockers (PCABs), specifically vonoprazan and Tegoprazan. PCABs are next-generation acid suppressants that inhibit the gastric H^+/K^+-ATPase (proton pump) in a potassium-competitive reversible manner. Its pharmacologic profile features a more rapid onset of action and a longer-lasting, more potent acid suppression than standard PPIs. In practical terms, vonoprazan can maintain intragastric pH >6 for extended periods even after a single dose, whereas PPIs often require several days to reach maximal effect and are limited by meal timing and CYP2C19 metabolism variability. The potent acid inhibition by PCABs creates a more favorable environment for antibiotics to work against *H. pylori* since *H. pylori* typically resides in the mucus layer and epithelial surface, which at high pH can be more easily penetrated by antibiotics.

Vonoprazan-based therapy was first approved in Japan and has shown impressive results in East Asian populations. For example, first-line vonoprazan triple therapy (vonoprazan + clarithromycin + amoxicillin for 7 days) demonstrated eradication rates of ~85–90%, which were significantly higher than those with a PPI-based triple therapy in the same studies [17, 18]. A 2022 meta-analysis of randomized trials found that overall, vonoprazan-based regimens were superior to PPI-based regimens in *H. pylori* eradication (pooled relative risk ~1.09, indicating a roughly 5–10% absolute improvement in cure rates) [18]. Notably, vonoprazan appears particularly beneficial in clarithromycin-resistant infections: some Japanese studies reported that vonoprazan-amoxicillin-clarithromycin triple therapy could still achieve ~80% eradication even when the strain was clarithromycin-resistant—a scenario where PPI triple therapy would usually fail. This is attributed to vonoprazan's strong acid suppression allowing amoxicillin to work more effectively and perhaps increasing clarithromycin's efficacy slightly despite resistance. Vonoprazan has also been utilized in dual therapy with just amoxicillin (taking advantage of the concept discussed earlier). A recent trial of 14-day vonoprazan + amoxicillin dual therapy in treatment-naïve patients achieved approximately 90% eradication, which was non-inferior to a vonoprazan triple regimen [15]. Such high-dose dual regimens with vonoprazan are promising because they simplify therapy and avoid macrolide or nitroimidazole use entirely, which is valuable in resistant populations.

Based on the accumulating evidence, regulatory approvals are expanding: vonoprazan-based therapies have now been approved in countries beyond Japan, including the United States (FDA approved a vonoprazan triple and a vonoprazan dual regimen in 2022 for *H. pylori* treatment). These approvals were supported by international phase III trials that showed the vonoprazan-clarithromycin-amoxicillin 14-day therapy was non-inferior to standard PPI triple therapy [19], with eradication rates around 80–85% even in regions with significant clarithromycin resistance. The vonoprazan-amoxicillin dual for 14 days also showed around 80% cure in one trial, providing an alternative for patients who cannot take clarithromycin. Vonoprazan's main side effects are similar to PPIs; it is generally well tolerated, though long-term use data are limited. The advent of vonoprazan marks an important tool to combat falling cure rates—by enhancing acid suppression, it essentially "turbocharges" existing antibiotic regimens. Many experts anticipate that PCAB-based regimens will replace PPI-based regimens in the coming years as first-line therapy in many areas, pending cost and availability, because of their higher barrier to resistance impact.

Another area of active development is new antibiotics or drug combinations. Research is ongoing into novel agents that could be used against *H. pylori*. One candidate under study is rifabutin in broader use (as mentioned, now formulated in a combination capsule for salvage therapy). Furazolidone, an older nitrofuran antibiotic, has seen renewed interest in regions where clarithromycin and metronidazole resistance are high; furazolidone-based quadruple therapies have shown good efficacy in China and the Middle East, though concerns about toxicity (it can cause systemic side effects at higher doses) limit its use. Nitazoxanide, another antiprotozoal drug, has been tested in place of metronidazole with some success. Moreover, adjunctive medications such as N-acetylcysteine to disrupt mucus or ecabet sodium (mucosal protectant) have been tried to improve antibiotic delivery to the gastric epithelium. These are not yet standard but exemplify attempts to improve treatment efficacy.

9. Non-pharmacological and adjunct approaches

While antibiotics are indispensable for eradicating *H. pylori*, various non-pharmacological or adjunct strategies have been explored to improve treatment outcomes or prevent infection. These include the use of probiotics, dietary and lifestyle modifications, as well as public health measures and vaccination efforts aimed at prevention.

Probiotics: Supplementation with probiotic organisms—typically strains of Lactobacillus, Bifidobacterium, Saccharomyces, and others—has been studied as an adjunct to *H. pylori* therapy. The rationale is that probiotics might inhibit *H. pylori* by several mechanisms: producing bacteriocins or acids that suppress *H. pylori*, competitively inhibiting its adhesion in the stomach, or modulating the host immune response to be less inflammatory. Additionally, probiotics are hypothesized to reduce antibiotic side effects like antibiotic-associated diarrhea and improve patient tolerance of therapy. A large number of randomized controlled trials have evaluated adding probiotics to standard triple or quadruple therapy. Meta-analyses indicate that probiotic supplementation can modestly increase *H. pylori* eradication rates and reduce treatment-related side effects [20]. For example, a recent network meta-analysis including 91 RCTs (over 13,000 patients) found that adding probiotics to standard therapy significantly improved eradication success (pooled eradication 78.8% with probiotics vs. 62.4% without, OR = 1.62) and also significantly decreased common side effects such as diarrhea (risk ratio ~0.5 for diarrhea with probiotics) [20]. The benefit appears more pronounced for certain probiotic strains; combinations of multiple strains may be more effective than single-strain supplements [20, 21]. The most evidence-supported strains include *Lactobacillus acidophilus*, *L. rhamnosus*, *Bifidobacterium bifidum*, *B. longum*, and the yeast *Saccharomyces boulardii*. While probiotics alone do not eradicate *H. pylori*, their adjunctive use is becoming a recommended practice to improve tolerability and possibly efficacy of antibiotic regimens. For instance, Maastricht VI consensus suggests considering probiotics to reduce side effects and increase compliance. It is important to note that not all studies show a large benefit—some trials have found no significant improvement—but overall the trend favors probiotic use, given their low risk. Typically, probiotics are started either 1–2 weeks before therapy or concurrently with the antibiotics and continued for the duration of treatment (and sometimes a couple weeks after). They are generally safe, with minimal adverse effects.

Diet and lifestyle modifications: Traditional advice for peptic ulcer patients included dietary modifications (bland diet, avoiding spices, etc.), but with the understanding that *H. pylori* is the root cause; diet per se is not a primary factor in ulcer disease. However, some dietary components may influence *H. pylori* colonization and gastritis severity. For example, diets high in salt have been shown in animal models to exacerbate *H. pylori*-induced gastric injury and increase risk of cancer; epidemiologically, high-salt intake correlates with gastric cancer risk in *H. pylori*-positive individuals. Thus, a low-salt diet might be prudent. Some foods contain compounds with anti-*H. pylori* activity: broccoli sprouts are rich in sulforaphane, which has been shown to inhibit *H. pylori* in vitro and in mice (small human studies suggest eating broccoli sprouts can transiently reduce urease output, an indicator of bacterial load). Green tea and cranberry juice have also demonstrated inhibitory effects in lab studies; a randomized trial found that regular cranberry juice consumption led to a modest reduction in *H. pylori* stool antigen positivity, hinting at a suppressive effect. Nonetheless, these are supplementary measures—none can reliably eradicate the infection alone. Moderating alcohol consumption and avoiding heavily pickled or smoked foods, which, along with *H. pylori*, synergistically increase gastric cancer risk are often recommended for infected individuals to protect the stomach lining.

A crucial lifestyle factor is avoiding NSAIDs (nonsteroidal anti-inflammatory drugs) or using them with caution. NSAIDs and *H. pylori* together exponentially increase the risk of peptic ulcer bleeding compared to either factor alone. In *H. pylori*-infected patients requiring long-term NSAIDs or aspirin, eradication of *H. pylori* is advised to lower ulcer risk. If *H. pylori* cannot be eradicated, prophylactic PPI therapy is indicated for those on NSAIDs. Smoking cessation is strongly recommended for infected individuals, since smoking impairs ulcer healing, promotes ulcer recurrence, and as noted earlier, may reduce the success of *H. pylori* therapy [9]. Quitting smoking not only helps the gastric mucosa heal but may also improve *H. pylori* eradication rates and decrease the likelihood of reinfection or ulcer relapse [22].

"Test-and-treat" strategy and mass eradication: From a public health perspective, strategies have been proposed to systematically identify and treat *H. pylori* infections to prevent disease. In healthcare settings, a common approach is test-and-treat for dyspepsia: non-invasive testing (urea breath test or stool antigen) is performed in patients with uninvestigated dyspeptic symptoms who are under 50 years old and have no alarming features; if positive, the patient is treated for *H. pylori*, and often symptoms improve [1]. This has become standard care in many countries because it can resolve symptoms and prevent ulcer disease without need for immediate endoscopy in young patients. Beyond individual care, some researchers advocate for population-wide *H. pylori* screening and treatment programs in regions at high risk for gastric cancer. For instance, in parts of East Asia with very high gastric cancer rates, modeling studies suggest that eradicating *H. pylori* in the population could substantially reduce cancer incidence over time. Community trials in China and Japan have demonstrated that mass eradication is feasible and can lead to a decline in precancerous lesions. However, concerns include cost, antibiotic resistance selection, and the logistics of identifying all carriers. In Japan, national policy now includes *H. pylori* testing and treatment for all citizens with chronic gastritis, aiming to eventually reduce gastric cancer burden. Similar pilot programs are underway in some high-incidence regions of China. These interventions treat *H. pylori* not just to alleviate current symptoms but as primary prevention of future disease, a testament to the importance of *H. pylori* as a public health target.

Vaccine: Developing a vaccine for *H. pylori* has long been seen as the ideal strategy for preventing infection or aiding eradication. Despite challenges posed by the bacterium's gastric niche and immune evasion, significant progress has been made. Both mucosal (oral/nasal) and parenteral vaccines have shown promise in animal models, with candidate antigens including urease subunits (UreA, UreB), CagA, VacA, flagellins, and adhesins like BabA [23, 24]. Therapeutic vaccines and improved formulations—using novel adjuvants (e.g., CpG, outer membrane vesicles) and delivery systems like nanoparticle—are under investigation. The ultimate goal is a childhood vaccine that confers lasting immunity, reducing reliance on antibiotics and potentially eliminating *H. pylori* infection globally.

Until an effective vaccine is widely available, prevention of *H. pylori* relies on general measures: improving sanitation, ensuring clean water, promoting hygiene (especially in food handling and within households to avoid oral transmission), and treating those infected to reduce the reservoir of contagion. Given *H. pylori*'s predominance in poorer regions, public health efforts that alleviate poverty and overcrowding are indirectly *H. pylori* prevention strategies as well. Interestingly, *H. pylori* prevalence has dropped in many countries as living standards have improved, even before specific medical interventions—reinforcing that economic development and hygiene are key components of controlling this infection.

In conclusion, the management of *H. pylori* infection is multifaceted—it involves effective antibiotic regimens tailored to overcome resistance, adjuvant measures to enhance success and tolerability, lifestyle modifications to reduce aggravating factors, and forward-looking strategies like vaccination for ultimate prevention.

The continuous rise in antibiotic resistance remains an ongoing challenge, necessitating updated treatment algorithms and investment in new diagnostics and therapeutics [4]. Nonetheless, with appropriate therapy, *H. pylori* can be cured in the vast majority of patients, leading to healing of gastritis and ulcers and significantly lowering the risks of gastric cancer and lymphoma. The discovery of *H. pylori* transformed our approach to peptic ulcer disease and gastric cancer—conditions once managed only palliatively can now be prevented by eradicating this bacterium [3]. As research progresses, the hope is to further reduce the global burden of *H. pylori* through optimized treatments and, eventually, vaccination, moving closer to a world where this "slow" bacterial infection no longer poses a threat to human health.

Author details

Arti Wongcha-Um[1], Tinpawee Thongkongthun[2]*, Ratha-korn Vilaichone[1] and Varocha Mahachai[1]

1 Chulabhorn International College of medicine, Excellence Center in Digestive Disease, Thammasat University, Pathum Thani, Thailand

2 Faculty of Medicine, Thammasat University, Pathum Thani, Thailand

*Address all correspondence to: iamvivieth@gmail.com

References

[1] Ahmad HM, Al-Fishawy HS, Shaltout I, Abd Elnaeem EA, Mohamed A. S, Salem AE. A comparative study between current and past *Helicobacter pylori* infection in terms of microalbuminuria in patients with type 2 diabetes. BMC Infectious Diseases. 2024;**24**(1), Article 1091. DOI: 10.1186/s12879-024-09918-5

[2] Yong X et al. *Helicobacter pylori* virulence factor CagA promotes tumorigenesis of gastric cancer via multiple signaling pathways. Cell Communication and Signaling: CCS. 2015;**13**:30. DOI: 10.1186/s12964-015-0111-0. Available from: https://pubmed.ncbi.nlm.nih.gov/26160167/

[3] Marshall B, Adams PC. *Helicobacter pylori*: A nobel pursuit? Canadian Journal of Gastroenterology. 2008;**22**(11):895-896. DOI: 10.1155/2008/459810. Available from: www.ncbi.nlm.nih.gov/pmc/articles/PMC2661189/

[4] Malfertheiner P et al. Management of *Helicobacter pylori* infection: The Maastricht VI/florence consensus report. Gut. 2022;**71**(9):1724-1762. DOI: *10.1136/gutjnl-2022-327745*

[5] Hooi JKY et al. Global prevalence of *Helicobacter pylori* infection: Systematic review and meta-analysis. Gastroenterology. 2017;**153**(2):420-429. DOI: 10.1053/j.gastro.2017.04.022

[6] Eusebi LH et al. Epidemiology of *Helicobacter pylori* infection. Helicobacter. 2014;**19**:1-5. DOI: 10.1111/hel.12165

[7] McMahon BJ et al. The diagnosis and treatment of *Helicobacter pylori* infection in arctic regions with a high prevalence of infection: Expert commentary. Epidemiology and Infection. 2015;**144**(2):225-233. DOI: 10.1017/s0950268815001181 [Accessed: November 4, 2021]

[8] World Health Organization, Regional Office for the Eastern Mediterranean. Role of *Helicobacter pylori* in the genesis of gastric ulcerations among smokers and nonsmokers. Vol. 3. No. 2. Cairo, Egypt: EMHJ; 2025. Available from: https://www.emro.who.int/emhj-volume-3-1997/volume-3-issue-2/article16.html

[9] Itskoviz D et al. Smoking increases the likelihood of *Helicobacter Pylori* treatment failure. Digestive and Liver Disease. 2017;**49**(7):764-768. DOI: 10.1016/j.dld.2017.03.010. Available from: www.sciencedirect.com/science/article/abs/pii/S1590865817307909 [Accessed: September 23, 2020]

[10] El-Omar EM et al. Interleukin-1 polymorphisms associated with increased risk of gastric cancer. Nature. 2000;**404**(6776):398-402. DOI: 10.1038/35006081. Available from: https://pubmed.ncbi.nlm.nih.gov/10746728/

[11] Owen RJ. Molecular testing for antibiotic resistance in *Helicobacter pylori*. Gut. 2002;**50**(3):285-289. DOI: 10.1136/gut.50.3.285 [Accessed: January 28, 2020]

[12] Pérez I et al. Management of *Helicobacter pylori* infection and effectiveness rates in daily clinical practice in Spain: 2010-2019. Antibiotics. 2022;**11**(5):698-698. DOI: 10.3390/antibiotics11050698 Accessed: August 21, 2023

[13] Öztürk K et al. High-dose dual therapy is effective as first-line treatment for *Helicobacter pylori* infection. The

Turkish Journal of Gastroenterology. 2020;**31**(3):234-238. DOI: 10.5152/tjg.2020.18974. Available from: www.ncbi.nlm.nih.gov/pmc/articles/PMC7197926/

[14] Yun J et al. The high-dose amoxicillin-proton pump inhibitor dual therapy in eradication of *Helicobacter pylori* infection. Expert Review of Gastroenterology & Hepatology. 2020;**15**(2):149-157. DOI: 10.1080/17474124.2021.1826306

[15] Yan T-L, Wang J-H, He X-J, Zhu Y-B, Lu L-J, Wang Y-J, et al. Ten-day vonoprazan–amoxicillin dual therapy vs. standard 14-day bismuth-based quadruple therapy for first-line *Helicobacter pylori* eradication: A multicenter randomized clinical trial. The American Journal of Gastroenterology. 2024;**119**(4):655-661. DOI: 10.14309/ajg.0000000000002592

[16] Yang E-H et al. 10-day versus 14-day bismuth quadruple therapy for first-line eradication of *Helicobacter pylori* infection: A randomised, open-label, non-inferiority trial. EClinicalMedicine. 2024;**70**:102529. DOI: 10.1016/j.eclinm.2024.102529

[17] Chen P-Y, Tsai F-P, Chen M-J, Yang H-Y, Wu M-S, Liou J-M. Vonoprazan-based versus proton pump inhibitor-based therapy in *Helicobacter pylori* eradication: An updated systematic review and meta-analysis of randomized trials. Gut. 2024;**73**(5):872-874. DOI: 10.1136/gutjnl-2023-329826

[18] Scarpignato C, Hunt RH. Potassium-competitive acid blockers: Current clinical use and future developments. Current Gastroenterology Reports. 2024;**26**(11):273-293. DOI: 10.1007/s11894-024-00939-3

[19] Fallone CA. The current role of vonoprazan in *Helicobacter pylori* treatment. Gastroenterology. 2022;**163**(3):572-574. DOI: 10.1053/j.gastro.2022.06.076 [Accessed: October 27, 2022]

[20] Tanashat M, Abuelazm M, Abouzid M, Al-Ajlouni YA, Ramadan A, Alsalah S, et al. Efficacy of probiotics regimens for *Helicobacter pylori* eradication: A systematic review, pairwise, and network meta-analysis of randomized controlled trials. Clinical Nutrition ESPEN. 2025;**65**:424-444. DOI: 10.1016/j.clnesp.2024.11.016

[21] Yang Z, Wang X, Li J, Chen Y, Zhang Q, Liu H. The effects of probiotics supplementation on *Helicobacter pylori* standard treatment: An umbrella review of systematic reviews with meta-analyses. Scientific Reports. 2024;**14**(1), Article 59399. DOI: 10.1038/s41598-024-59399-4

[22] Johns Hopkins Medicine. Smoking and the Digestive System. 2024. Available from: www.hopkinsmedicine.org/health/conditions-and-diseases/smoking-and-the-digestive-system

[23] Yunle K et al. Advances in *Helicobacter pylori* vaccine research: From candidate antigens to adjuvants—A review. Helicobacter. 2024;**29**(1):e13034. Available from: https://pubmed.ncbi.nlm.nih.gov/37971157/. DOI: 10.1111/hel.13034

[24] Zeng M et al. Efficacy, safety, and immunogenicity of an oral recombinant *Helicobacter pylori* vaccine in children in China: A randomised, double-blind, placebo-controlled, phase 3 trial. The Lancet. 2015;**386**(10002):1457-1464. DOI: 10.1016/S0140-6736(15)60310-5. Available from: https://reader.elsevier.com/reader/sd/pii/S0140673615603105?token=7FF9D938086422E05AC6D9777AD523EA81CD8FC1597A2DF1605AA382D41AC08532DB8801B8F9A1A1D3ED5998C96C1FB7

Chapter 3

Helicobacter pylori Infection: Routine and Molecular Strategies for Diagnosing *Helicobacter pylori* in the New Era

Qingsheng Liu, Suting Qian, Haoyu Zhao, Chuying Yu and Xintong Ye

Abstract

Helicobacter pylori (*Hp*) infection remains a prevalent global health concern associated with significant gastrointestinal (GI) morbidity. Current diagnostic approaches encompass both invasive (endoscopy with histology/culture) and non-invasive (urea breath test (UBT)) methodologies. However, rising antibiotic resistance has substantially compromised empirical eradication therapies, necessitating advanced diagnostic solutions. Emerging molecular techniques demonstrate superior diagnostic performance, including polymerase chain reaction (PCR)-based assays, next-generation sequencing (NGS), and DNA microarrays. Innovative platforms, such as matrix-assisted laser desorption/ionization-time-of-flight mass spectrometry (MALDI-TOF MS), enable rapid *H. pylori* identification and antibiotic resistance profiling directly from clinical samples. Particularly noteworthy is ultrasensitive chromosomal aneuploidy detection (UCAD) technology, which provides comprehensive genomic analysis for precise resistance mutation detection through high-throughput whole-genome sequencing (WGS). These technological advances promise to revolutionize *H. pylori* management in the era of increasing antimicrobial resistance.

Keywords: *Helicobacter pylori*, diagnosis, traditional methods, molecular techniques, antibiotic resistance

1. Introduction

Helicobacter pylori (*H. pylori*), a Gram-negative bacterium colonizing the human gastric mucosa, is a well-established etiological agent for chronic gastritis, peptic ulcers, gastric mucosa-associated lymphoid tissue (MALT) lymphoma, and gastric adenocarcinoma [1]. Despite declining prevalence in developed nations [2], global infection rates remain substantial (>50% in adults), with marked variations across geographic regions, age groups, ethnicities, and socioeconomic strata [3]. The bacterium's virulence factors (e.g., vacuolating cytotoxin A (VacA), cytotoxin-associated gene A (CagA), induced by contact with epithelium gene A (IceA)) induce gastric epithelial damage through well-characterized mechanisms [4], prompting their classification as a Group 1 carcinogen by the International Agency for Research on Cancer (IARC). Crucially, *H. pylori* eradication significantly reduces gastric cancer risk, forming a global therapeutic consensus [5]. Therefore, early diagnosis and effective treatment of *Hp* infection are important for the prevention of chronic gastritis, peptic ulcer, and even gastric cancer. Notably, *Hp* detection is a key link to achieve this goal. Based on clinical practice, this article systematically reviews the worldwide research progress in *Hp*, summarizes the advantages and limitations of current conventional *Hp* detection methods, and explores the great potential of future molecular detection strategies in *Hp* diagnosis, with a view to providing references and new ideas to improve the accuracy of *Hp* detection.

2. Routine diagnosis of *H. pylori*

Current diagnostic methods for *H. pylori* infection are broadly classified into invasive and non-invasive approaches. Invasive techniques require endoscopic biopsy followed by histological examination, rapid urease testing, or culture. While offering high specificity and enabling antibiotic susceptibility testing, their invasive nature limits patient acceptance. Non-invasive alternatives, including the urea breath test (UBT), stool antigen tests, and serological assays, provide convenient, rapid, and cost-effective options suitable for initial diagnosis and post-treatment monitoring. However, these methods exhibit variable sensitivity and specificity due to susceptibility to multiple confounding factors. The following sections detail the technical aspects, advantages, and limitations of each diagnostic modality.

2.1 Invasive methods

2.1.1 Endoscopy

Endoscopic evaluation was performed according to the Kyoto Classification of Gastritis [6], incorporating 19 standardized findings. Key diagnostic features included: mucosal atrophy, intestinal metaplasia, fold enlargement, nodularity, diffuse redness, and regular arrangement of collecting venules (RAC) (**Table 1**). A Kyoto gastritis score of ≥ 2 is highly suggestive of *Hp* infection.

Advantages: 1. High diagnostic accuracy: a Kyoto score ≥ 2 predicts *H. pylori* infection with 90% accuracy [7]. Endoscopic features, such as nodular gastritis and regularly arranged RACs, can significantly improve the diagnostic accuracy [8, 9]. 2. Intuitive assessment of lesions: endoscopy can directly observe the lesion area of gastric mucosa, which helps to assess the degree of gastric mucosal inflammation, atrophy, intestinal metaplasia, and other lesions, and to further determine the risk of gastric cancer. 3. Multi-dimensional detection support: samples obtained by endoscopy can be used for pathogenetic Detection and histological examination, which not only improves the diagnostic accuracy, but also provides drug sensitivity experimental data support for follow-up treatment and guides individualized treatment plan.

Limitations: 1. Limitations of invasive operation: endoscopy is an invasive operation, the acceptance of patients is generally low, which may affect the compliance of the examination due to discomfort or fear. 2. Influence of subjectivity: the observation of endoscopic manifestations is highly subjective, and the completion of an

Endoscopic findings	Score
Atrophy	
None–C1	0
C2–C3	1
O1–O3	2
Intestinal metaplasia	
None	0
Antrum	1
Corpus and antrum	2
Enlarged folds	
No	0
Yes	1
Nodular gastritis	
No	0
Yes	1
Erythema diffusion	
None	0
Mild (with RAC)	1
Severe	2
Kyoto score	0–8

Table 1.
Kyoto classification score.

accurate diagnosis of *Hp* infection by relying on the endoscopic manifestations alone is highly dependent on the endoscopist's technical level and clinical experience, and therefore, it is necessary to combine with histological examination and pathogenetic testing to improve the accuracy of diagnosis.

2.1.2 Histological examination

Procedure: As many as 2–3 pieces of biopsy tissue need to be obtained from sites, such as the gastric antrum and gastric body [10]. Subsequently, the obtained biopsy tissues were fixed, dehydrated, embedded, and sectioned into thin slices of 4–5 μm thickness. Next, the processed biopsy samples were stained and observed under a microscope. Commonly used staining methods include conventional hematoxylin-eosin (HE) staining, Giemsa staining, Warthin-Starry silver staining, and immuno-histochemical staining. In clinical practice, HE staining usually meets the diagnostic needs of routine *Hp* infection. However, in cases of moderate to severe gastritis or unsatisfactory HE staining results, ancillary staining methods are recommended. Immunohistochemical staining and Giemsa staining are the preferred auxiliary staining methods in clinical practice [11, 12].

Advantages: Histological examination remains the gold standard for *H. pylori* diagnosis, maintaining its primary role in clinical practice [13]. This method offers two key advantages: exceptional specificity for bacterial detection, and concurrent evaluation of gastritis severity and precancerous lesions when combined with endoscopic findings. The combined histo-endoscopic approach enables comprehensive disease assessment, guiding optimal clinical management decisions.

Limitations: 1. Interfering factors: the use of proton pump inhibitors (PPIs) and antibiotics may interfere with the test results, therefore, patients are advised to discontinue antibiotics and PPIs for at least 2 weeks prior to the test [13]. 2. Sample error: due to the limited extent of the biopsy site, it may lead to false-negative results. Therefore, in histologic testing, it is usually necessary to obtain 2–3 pieces of biopsy tissue from different sites to improve diagnostic accuracy [14].

2.1.3 Rapid urease test (RUT)

Procedure: The biopsy sample obtained by gastroscopy is put into the medium containing urea and pH indicator. Urease produced by *Hp* hydrolyzes urea to ammonia, resulting in a change in pH, which changes the color of the reagent from yellow to red or pink.

Advantages: 1. Rapidity: the results are usually obtained within a few minutes to 24 hours, which is suitable for rapid clinical diagnosis. 2. Simplicity: the operation process is simple, the cost of reagents is low, and no complex equipment is required, which is easy to popularize the application at all levels of health care institutions. 3. High specificity: the current commercial RUT reagents have high sensitivity and specificity, in which the specificity is even as high as 98.3–100% [15], and the test results are reliable, and the detection results are reliable. In addition, studies have shown that the diagnostic accuracy can be improved by increasing the number of biopsy samples, which helps to correct the sampling error due to the uneven distribution of *H. pylori* [16, 17].

Limitations: 1. Interfering factors: low bacterial load, recent use of acid-suppressing drugs or antibiotics may lead to false-negative results [13, 18]. Therefore, a longer period of drug withdrawal than histologic testing is required before performing RUT. Second, in patients with gastrointestinal bleeding, RUT may show false-positive results due to the interference of alkaline substances in the blood, thus affecting clinical judgment [19]. 2. Inability to assess histopathology: RUT can only detect the presence of *Hp*, and it cannot provide information about the pathology of the gastric mucosa, which limits its clinical value to a certain extent.

2.1.4 Bacterial culture

Procedure: Gastric mucosal biopsy samples obtained by gastroscopy were inoculated in selective medium. The samples were incubated at 35–37°C for at least 5–7 days in a microaerobic environment. At the end of the incubation, the surface of the medium is observed and *Hp* is confirmed by biochemical tests, such as Gram staining, oxidase test, urease test, etc. Generally, *Hp* colonies are clear or grayish-white, with a diameter of 1–2 mm. On the basis of this morphology, combined with the positive urease, catalase, and oxidase reactions, and Gram-negative biochemical characteristics, the diagnosis of *Hp* infection can be made.

Advantages: 1. High specificity: culture method is the gold standard for the diagnosis of *H. pylori* infection, the specificity is almost 100%, it can accurately identify the pathogenic bacteria, and provide a reliable basis for clinical diagnosis. 2. Drug sensitivity test: antibiotic sensitivity test can be performed after culture, which can guide the clinic in choosing the optimal treatment plan, especially in the areas or populations where the primary resistance rate of Clarithromycin is higher than 15%, the culture of *Hp* and drug sensitivity test are important for the optimization of treatment strategy and reduction of drug-resistance risk. Optimize treatment strategies and reduce the risk of drug resistance [13]. 3. Strain preservation: culture can isolate preserved *H. pylori* strains and provide resources for subsequent studies, such as genetic analysis, virulence factor studies, and epidemiological investigations.

Limitations: 1. Low sensitivity: the sensitivity of the culture method is susceptible to a variety of factors, including the use of acid-suppressing drugs and antibiotics, the mode of sample transfer, culture conditions, and bias in sampling location. Therefore, similar to RUT and histology, it is important to ensure that the patient is off acid-suppressing drugs and antibiotics for at least 2 weeks before performing culture. In addition, to improve the sensitivity of the culture method, two tissue samples should be taken from each of the gastric antrum and the gastric body during gastroscopy [20, 21]. 2. Time-consuming: culture takes 5–7 days, which lacks timeliness and may affect immediate clinical decision-making. 3. High culture transit conditions: *H. pylori* is extremely sensitive to the culture environment, and delays in transportation or exposure of samples to aerobic environments may lead to bacterial Delay in transportation or exposure of samples to aerobic environment may lead to bacterial inactivation, thus affecting the accuracy of culture results [22].

2.2 Non-invasive methods

2.2.1 Urea breath test (UBT)

Procedure: Patients need to stop taking antibiotics and PPIs for at least 2 weeks before the test and remain fasting for more than 6 hours on the day of the test. The test begins with a baseline sample of the patient's exhaled breath. Subsequently, a ^{13}C- or ^{14}C-labeled urea solution is taken and the exhaled gas is collected again as a test sample after waiting for 15–30 minutes. Finally, a mass spectrometer or scintillation counter is used to detect the amount of labeled CO_2 in the sample. If the concentration of labeled CO_2 in the test sample is significantly higher than that in the baseline sample, it is determined to be *Hp* positive.

Advantages: 1. Highly accurate: UBT detects *Hp* urease activity and labels the CO_2 produced by the breakdown of urea, which makes the results more objective, highly sensitive, and specific, with remarkable diagnostic accuracy [23, 24]. 2. Widely applicable: UBT is easy to perform, non-invasive, and reproducible, and the results can be obtained in a few hours, which makes it suitable for the initial screening of *Hp*, the evaluation of the efficacy of eradication therapy, and the screening of children for *Hp* screening [13, 25].

Limitations: 1. High number of interfering factors: the use of PPIs and antibiotics, gastrointestinal bleeding, and atypical pathogen infections may affect the accuracy of UBT results [26, 27]. 2. Radiological risk: ^{14}C-labeled urea is slightly radioactive and therefore not suitable for use in children and pregnant women. ^{13}C does not have any associated pitfalls. 3. Cost and equipment requirements: UBT testing relies on specific equipment and is expensive, factors that limit its popularity in remote and economically underdeveloped areas. 4. The optimal timing and the optimal critical level of UBT have not been fully determined, which may have some impact on the accuracy of the test [28].

2.2.2 Stool antigen test (SAT)

Procedure: Fresh stool samples were collected from patients and mixed with the extract. Subsequently, the supernatant is centrifuged and tested for *Hp* antigens in the supernatant using an enzyme-linked immunosorbent assay (ELISA) or immunochromatographic assay (ICA). The results of the test are determined by observing a color change or measuring the signal intensity, with a positive result indicating the presence of infection and a negative result indicating no sign of infection.

Advantages: 1. High sensitivity and specificity: relevant meta-analysis showed that the sensitivity and specificity of SAT were as high as 94% and 97%, respectively, and could accurately detect *Hp* infection [29], and the most recommended SAT assay in clinical practice is monoclonal ELISA. 2. Widely applicable: like UBT, SAT is also applicable to the first-time diagnosis, efficacy evaluation of eradication therapy [30–33]. 3. Inexpensive: Compared with UBT, SAT does not require the support of appropriate equipment and is inexpensive, making it more suitable for large-scale screening.

Limitations: More interfering factors: similar to UBT, the accuracy of SAT is affected by a variety of factors, including stool shape, antibiotic and PPI medication history, N-acetylcysteine, and GI bleeding [34]. In addition, temperature, transit time, and storage conditions can have an impact on the results [35].

2.2.3 Serological test

Procedure: Draw patient's venous blood and separate serum, add serum to the kit and incubate at the appropriate temperature, wash the unbound antigen-antibody after incubation, add color developer, and finally read the level of immunoglobulin G (IgG) antibody to *Hp* by colorimetry or instrumentation.

Advantages: 1. Low cost: the serological test is cheap and rapid, suitable for epidemiological studies and large-scale screening. 2. Low interference: its accuracy is not affected by factors, such as GI bleeding, history of PPI and antibiotic use, or gastric mucosal atrophy. 3. It can be used in combination with biomarkers to identify high-risk patients: the evaluation system of pepsinogen (PG) I, PG II, and PG I/II ratio in conjunction with the *Hp* antibody is widely used to assess the risk of atrophic gastritis and gastric cancer [13, 36]; in addition, antibodies to virulence factors CagA, VacA, and *Escherichia coli* chaperone protein (GroEL) can be used as potential predictors of high-risk strains [37–39].

Limitations: 1. Geographical variation: the accuracy of serologic testing varies regionally depending on the prevalence of antigens and specific *H. pylori* strains [40], and reagent selection needs to be adapted to locally prevalent strains. 2. Inability to differentiate between presenting and previous infections: antibody levels persist long after *Hp* eradication, and therefore serologic testing is not indicated for post-treatment follow-up [13].

3. Novel molecular diagnostic method of *H. pylori*

With the increase in antibiotic resistance and a significant rise in the failure rate of traditional empirical eradication therapies, molecular diagnostic methods have gained much attention due to their high sensitivity, specificity, and ability to detect markers of antibiotic resistance.

3.1 Polymerase chain reaction (PCR)

Procedure: The DNA of *Hp* is extracted from gastric biopsy samples, feces, or saliva and purified to remove proteins and other impurities. Specific primers are designed to target *Hp*-specific genes. The PCR system was configured, including DNA template, specific primers, deoxynucleotide triphosphates (dNTPs), Taq DNA polymerase, buffer, and Mg^{2+}. Amplification was performed under specific conditions using a PCR instrument. The amplified products are analyzed by agarose gel electrophoresis or real-time fluorescent quantitative PCR (qPCR) [41–43].

Advantages: 1. High sensitivity and specificity: PCR has high sensitivity and specificity, which can be seen in the detection of very low concentrations of *Hp* DNA, and the sensitivity and specificity of some nested PCRs can even be up to 100% [44, 45], so properly executed nested PCRs were once regarded as the new gold standard for *Hp* detection [46]. 2. Drug-resistance genes detection: PCR can simultaneously detect the drug-resistance genes of *Hp*, such as ureA [47], Hsp60 [44], and clarithromycin resistance gene 23S rRNA [48], providing guidance for personalized treatment. 3. Multiple specimen types: PCR is applicable to a wide range of samples, such as gastric mucosal tissues, feces, saliva, etc., to satisfy different clinical needs [41].

Limitations: 1. Risk of contamination: PCR is very sensitive to contamination, and very small amounts of exogenous DNA may lead to false-positive results, which requires strict operational specifications [49]. 2. Cost and technical threshold: DNA extraction, reaction system configuration, and result analysis require professional technicians to operate, and the technical threshold is high. In addition, PCR requires specialized instruments with high cost. 3. Primer design challenges: The primer design link is related to the sensitive new and specificity of the results, which needs to be repeatedly verified and optimized. 4. Unable to distinguish between live and dead bacteria: Because PCR directly detects the DNA of *Hp*, it is unable to distinguish whether the *Hp* is live or dead, which may lead to a false-positive result after treatment.

3.2 Fluorescence in situ hybridization (FISH)

Procedure: Tissue sections of gastroscopic biopsy samples are processed, followed by designing complementary fluorescent-labeled probes targeting *Hp*-specific gene sequences and binding them to DNA or RNA molecules on the sections. Unbound probes are removed during the washing step and the fluorescent signal is detected by fluorescence microscopy to achieve confirmation of the presence of *H. pylori* [50].

Advantages: 1. High sensitivity and specificity: commercially available FISH assays have a sensitivity of 90–97% and specificity of 94–100% for *Hp* detection [51, 52], which can meet the needs of early diagnosis. 2. Direct observation: bacteria in tissues can be observed directly by fluorescence microscopy, avoiding DNA contamination and the interference of dead strains [53]. 3. Detection of drug-resistant mutations: FISH. By designing specific fluorescent probes, the mutation sites of drug-resistance genes can be targeted, and the results have high sensitivity and specificity [54], especially in the detection of clarithromycin resistance, which is more reliable and sensitive than the conventional drug sensitivity test [50].

Limitations: 1. Invasive: FISH testing still requires gastroscopic biopsy specimens, which is an invasive operation with low patient acceptance. 2. Cost and technology threshold: FISH testing relies on fluorescence microscopy, probes, and reagents, which make the testing expensive. 3. Time-consuming: From sample processing to result analysis, FISH testing usually takes several hours to days, which is not able to meet the demand for rapid diagnosis.

3.3 Next-generation sequencing (NGS)

Procedure: Samples for NGS can be derived from biopsy tissue, feces, saliva, or gastric fluid. Following sample lysis and total DNA extraction, molecular analysis proceeds via either targeted sequencing (PCR amplification of specific genes) or whole-genome sequencing (DNA fragmentation and adapter ligation). After high-throughput sequencing using Illumina or Nanopore platforms, data quality control, sequence comparison, identification of resistance mutations and virulence genes, and ultimately generation of analysis reports are used to guide the clinic [55, 56].

Advantages: 1. Comprehensiveness: simultaneous detection of multiple genetic variants provides more complete genetic information, which is significantly better than traditional drug sensitivity tests or single-gene PCR [57–59]. 2. High sensitivity: detection of low-abundance mutations is more sensitive than traditional methods, and is suitable for mixed infection analysis [60]. 3. Wide range of research potentials: supports strain evolution analysis, chain of transmission tracking, and drug-resistance prediction, providing an Epidemiologic investigation that provides efficient tools [61, 62].

Limitations: 1. Cost and technical threshold: rely on expensive sequencing equipment and require professional bioinformatics team for data analysis. 2. Poor timeliness: from sample to result takes 2–5 days, which is not as timely as the traditional detection methods. 3. DNA contamination and interference from dead bacteria: similar to PCR, NGS, as a class of DNA-based technology, is susceptible to contamination, and it is not able to identify the interference from dead bacteria [63]. NGS is similar to PCR, in that it is susceptible to contamination and cannot recognize interference from dead bacteria [63].

3.4 CRISPR-based diagnostics

Procedure: Following extraction of DNA/RNA from clinical specimens (e.g., biopsy tissue, feces, saliva, or blood), target sequences may be amplified when enhanced sensitivity is required. Subsequently, a *H. pylori*-specific crRNA (CRISPR (clustered regularly interspaced palindromic repeats) RNA) is designed and complexed with Cas proteins and reporter molecules to establish the detection system, with results visualized through fluorescence emission or lateral flow strip colorimetric changes [64, 65].

Advantages: 1. High sensitivity and specificity: Based on the precise recognition of crRNA, the CRISPR-Cas (clustered regularly interspaced palindromic repeats-CRISPR-associated protein 9) system can differentiate *H. pylori* subtypes and drug-resistant mutations, with a detection limit as low as 2–10 copies/μL, which is significantly better than conventional molecular detection methods in terms of sensitivity and specificity [66–68]. 2. Convenient and fast: Without complicated instruments, the lateral flow chromatography test strip method can even achieve visual interpretation, and is much faster than conventional molecular detection methods. Detection can be completed within 30 minutes, much faster than culture method and qPCR [69]. 3. Lower cost: Compared with qPCR and NGS technology, CRISPR technology does not require the support of expensive equipment and reagents, which is suitable for grassroots applications. 4. Multi-targeted detection: Multi-crRNAs can be designed to synchronously detect pathogens, virulence genes, and drug-resistance mutations, which improves the diagnostic efficiency [70].

Limitations: 1. Standardization challenge: Currently, CRISPR diagnostic technology has not yet formed a unified operational standard, and the testing process of different laboratories varies, which affects the comparability of results. 2. Inhibitor interference: Inhibitors in clinical samples may reduce the activity of the CRISPR system, resulting in false-negative results, and sample processing methods need to be optimized [71]. 3. Ethical issues: The gene-editing capabilities could be misused, and a regulatory framework is needed to ensure that it is only used in compliant medical diagnostics [72].

3.5 DNA microarray

Procedure: DNA microarray detection utilizes PCR-amplified target sequences incorporating fluorescent-labeled nucleotides, which are subsequently hybridized with chip-immobilized probes; the resulting hybridization patterns are then scanned and analyzed to generate comprehensive reports detailing *H. pylori* infection status, antibiotic resistance profiles, and virulence factor expression patterns [73].

Advantages: 1. Multi-gene detection: Simultaneous analysis of virulence genes, drug resistance, and strain typing significantly improves the diagnostic efficiency compared with traditional PCR or culture methods, which is suitable for the diagnosis of difficult cases or epidemiological studies. 2. High sensitivity and specificity: The detection limit of the DNA microarray assay reaches 102 copies/μL [74, 75], and the sensitivity is greater than 95% [76]. Specificity is optimized by probe design to reduce cross-reactivity [77, 78]. 3. Rapid and automated: the whole process is completed in 6–8 hours, and automated analysis reduces human error and time loss [74, 76].

Limitations: 1. High cost and technical threshold: expensive microarray preparation and scanning equipment are required, and the analysis is dependent on specialized personnel, thus limiting clinical dissemination. 2. Cross-contamination and dead bacterial interference: PCR cross-contamination may interfere with the results, and there is no way to distinguish between live/dead bacteria, so it is not applicable to the assessment of efficacy after eradication therapy [79].

3.6 Matrix-assisted laser desorption/ionization-time-of-flight mass spectrometry (MALDI-TOF MS)

Procedure: MALDI-TOF MS enables rapid detection of *H. pylori* from diverse clinical specimens (gastric mucosa, gastric juice, feces, blood, and urine) through a standardized workflow involving microbial colony isolation, target plate spotting with matrix solution to form co-crystals, laser-induced ionization, and time-of-flight separation of protein/peptide ions by mass-to-charge ratio (m/z); spectral peaks are then compared against reference databases, with a matching score ≥ 2.0 indicating reliable identification while simultaneously detecting resistance-associated protein variants [80, 81].

Advantages: 1. Rapid and efficient: the assay can be completed in 10–30 minutes, and the simultaneous identification of species, typing, and drug-resistance analysis can be realized, which is significantly more efficient than the traditional culture and PCR methods [81, 82]. 2. High sensitivity and specificity: the lowest limit of detection reaches 10^4–10^6 CFU/mL, and the cross-reactivity is avoided by the characteristic protein profiles, which ensures the accuracy of the results [83, 84]. 3. Low consumables and automation: less consumables are required and the fully automated process effectively reduces human error. Multi-sample compatibility: compatible with all types of clinical samples and mixed flora analysis [85–87].

Limitations: 1. High sample processing requirements: pre-purification and culture of colonies are required, which prolong the detection cycle, and in vitro culture of *Hp* is difficult [88]. 2. Database dependence: rare or variant strains may be missed due to insufficient database coverage [89]. 3. High equipment and technical threshold:

mass spectrometers are costly and require specialized personnel to operate and perform regular maintenance. 4. Interference of dead bacteria: only protein signals are detected, and it is impossible to distinguish between live/dead bacteria, so it is not applicable to live/dead bacteria.

3.7 Ultrasensitive chromosomal aneuploidy detection (UCAD)

Procedure: UCAD using body fluid free DNA or tissue genomic DNA as a template, chromosomal instability of the examinee is detected at the genome-wide level through low coverage whole-genome sequencing (LC-WGS), combined with bioinformatics analysis, to achieve qualitative and quantitative detection of chromosomal stability.

Advantages: This high-throughput detection system demonstrates exceptional accuracy (sensitivity of 1:1000 for single tests and 1:1,000,000 for repeated tests), broad applicability across diverse sample types (peripheral blood, exfoliated cells, menstrual blood, fresh/frozen/FFPE (formalin-fixed paraffin-embedded) tissues, and urine), and comprehensive diagnostic capabilities encompassing detection of various malignancies, identification of drug-resistant mutations, and characterization of antibiotic resistance profiles while providing complete genetic information.

Limitations: 1. High costs associated with whole-genome sequencing (WGS) and subsequent data analysis compared to conventional methods; 2. requirement for sophisticated bioinformatics pipelines encompassing sequence alignment, copy number variation (CNV) detection, and statistical modeling; 3. dependence on sample DNA quality where compromised samples (e.g., low-abundance cell-free DNA in liquid biopsies) may yield false-positive or false-negative results; and 4. insufficient validation in large-scale clinical cohorts to establish robust performance metrics.

4. Emerging trends and future directions of *H. pylori*

4.1 Prompt onset testing (POCT)

POCT technology refers to the testing technology in the clinic with the core features of rapidity, convenience, and simplicity of operation. In recent years, POCT technology has made significant progress under the impetus of multidisciplinary cross-fertilization. It is mainly reflected in the following levels:

4.1.1 Innovation of technology platform

1. Microfluidics and lab-on-a-chip: Microfluidic chip technology realizes significant simplification of the testing process through highly integrated sample processing, reaction, and detection modules. Its fully automated design not only significantly reduces the consumption of samples and reagents, but also effectively avoids cross-contamination and manual errors, and truly achieves the integrated detection of "sample in—result out." At present, this technology has shown outstanding application potential in the fields of *Hp* nucleic acid detection, specific antibody screening, and drug-resistant gene mutation analysis, providing rapid and accurate testing solutions for clinical practice [90–92].

2. Molecular diagnostic POCT: The breakthrough development of isothermal amplification technology enables nucleic acid amplification to completely get rid of the dependence on PCR instrument and significantly shorten the amplification time [93]. The combination of this technology with a digital microfluidic (DMF) system can synchronize the detection of *Hp* conserved genes and virulence genes within 30 minutes with a sensitivity of up to 10 copies/mL [94]. More notably, the coupling of isothermal amplification with the CRISPR-Cas system further enhanced the detection performance, demonstrating excellent specificity and sensitivity in *Hp* detection while keeping the total detection time within 40 minutes. These innovative technologies have significantly improved the timeliness of molecular diagnosis and provided new solutions for rapid and accurate diagnosis of *Hp* infection [68].

3. Biosensors: Optical sensors such as surface plasmon resonance (SPR), fluorescent labeling, and other technologies as well as the application of nano-enhanced materials can dramatically improve the sensitivity of molecular detection. It enables conventional molecular techniques to get rid of the defects of bulky and expensive detection equipment [95, 96].

4.1.2 Clinical optimization

POCT technology is rapidly developing toward multi-target integrated detection and intelligent application. Modern platforms have realized the simultaneous detection of pathogen nucleic acids, antibodies, virulence factors, and resistance genes, combined with diversified sample collection and smartphone AI interpretation, making accurate home testing possible. These breakthroughs are driving the transformation of POCT into a "home laboratory" model, significantly improving clinical testing efficiency and application scope.

4.1.3 Performance improvement

POCT technology with its high accuracy, rapid detection, and low-cost advantages shows significant development potential. Currently, the detection sensitivity of mainstream POCT products generally exceeds 90%, and the detection time can be controlled within 20–30 minutes, while the detection cost is only about 40% of the traditional PCR technology [97–99].

4.2 Microbiome analysis

H. pylori profoundly modifies the gastric microenvironment through urease secretion, virulence factor release, and induction of localized inflammation [100]. These alterations not only disrupt indigenous microbial communities but also facilitate the formation of polymicrobial biofilms that enable symbiotic relationships with other gastric microorganisms. Intriguingly, this symbiosis exhibits bidirectional regulation: while certain probiotics suppress *H. pylori* growth via antimicrobial production, membrane disruption, and competitive mucosal adhesion [101], oral-derived bacteria enhance its gastric colonization, and some resident gastric species even provide essential nutrients [102–105]. Furthermore, specific microbes promote *H. pylori* persistence by modulating host immunity to reduce bacterial clearance or augment antibiotic resistance, highlighting the complex ecological interactions governing *H. pylori* pathogenesis [100, 106].

These findings have important clinical implications. Meanwhile, a large number of studies have shown that the interaction between *Hp* and the gastric microbiota is closely related to the development of several gastric diseases [107]. This suggests that an in-depth analysis of the gastric microbiome may not only provide new biomarkers in diagnosis and disease risk assessment, but may also provide an important basis for the development of novel therapeutic strategies based on microbiome modulation. In the future, a new paradigm of "ecological-immune" integrated diagnosis and treatment is expected to be established through the integration of innovative technologies, such as *Hp*-targeted clearance, precise microbiome regulation, and host immune microenvironment modulation, which is more efficient and more personalized.

4.3 Artificial intelligence (AI)

AI has made significant progress in the field of *Hp* diagnosis, dramatically improving the accuracy, sensitivity, and timeliness of diagnosis by integrating endoscopic image analysis, pathology detection, and molecular biology techniques.

In endoscopic diagnosis, AI analyzes gastroscopy images based on deep learning algorithms, which can efficiently identify mucosal features of *Hp* infection. Several multi-center studies have confirmed that the accuracy rate of endoscopy-assisted diagnosis system using convolutional neural network (CNN) is more than 90% [108–109], which significantly improves the diagnostic level of endoscopists.

In the field of pathology detection, AI can accurately identify the morphology and distribution of *Hp* by analyzing the stained images of gastric mucosa biopsy sections. The deep learning AI algorithm can increase the detection sensitivity to 95–100% [110, 111], further optimize the diagnostic performance by combining with digital pathology scanning technology [112], and significantly reduce the workload of pathologists.

In molecular biology testing, AI improves the accuracy of critical value determination by optimizing the data analysis of UBT. In addition, the combination of AI and immunochromatography significantly improved the automation level and sensitivity of SAT, making it more suitable for primary care [113].

In the future, the development of AI will focus on multimodal data integration to provide personalized diagnosis and treatment plans for patients. Diagnostic devices are evolving toward portability and wearability, and AI-based studies of gastric microecology and *Hp* interactions will open new avenues for novel biomarker discovery.

5. Conclusion

The diagnosis of *H. pylori* infection continues to evolve with advances in both conventional and molecular techniques. While conventional methods are still widely used, molecular diagnostic strategies offer greater sensitivity, specificity, and the ability to detect antibiotic resistance, paving the way for personalized treatment (**Figure 1**). The integration of emerging technologies, such as immediate detection, microbiome analysis, and artificial intelligence, is expected to further improve diagnostic accuracy and patient prognosis in the new era of *H. pylori* management.

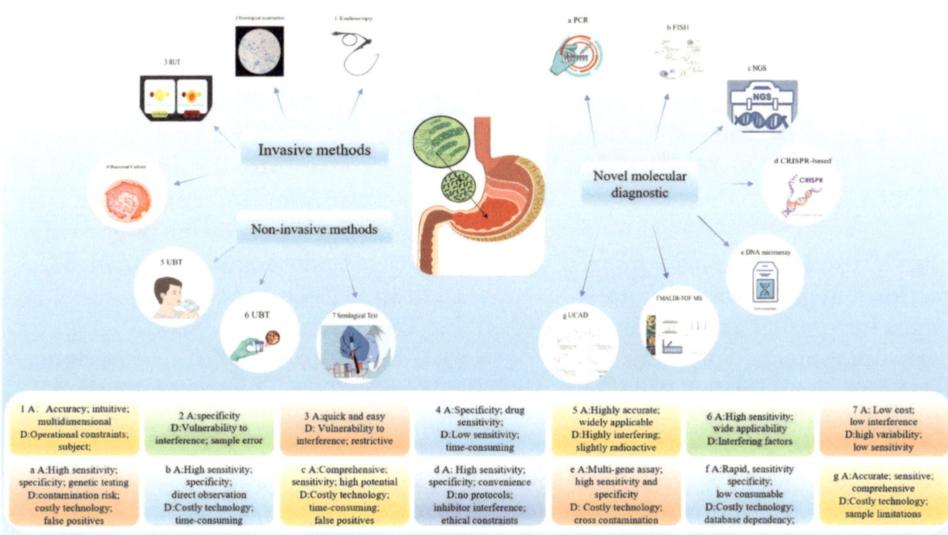

Figure 1.
Routine and molecular strategies for diagnosing Hp.

Acknowledgements

We gratefully acknowledge the kind cooperation of all authors in the preparation of this paper.

Conflict of interest

The authors declare no conflict of interest.

Author details

Qingsheng Liu*, Suting Qian, Haoyu Zhao, Chuying Yu and Xintong Ye
Department of Digestive, Hangzhou Hospital of TCM Affiliated to Zhejiang Chinese Medical University, Hangzhou, Zhejiang, China

*Address all correspondence to: 7394822@qq.com

References

[1] Dunn BE, Cohen H, Blaser MJ. *Helicobacter pylori*. Clinical Microbiology Reviews. 1997;**10**:720-741. DOI: 10.1128/CMR.10.4.720

[2] Pan Y, Jiao F. *Helicobacter pylori* infection and gastric microbiota: Insights into gastric and duodenal ulcer development. World Journal of Gastroenterology. 2025;**31**:100044. DOI: 10.3748/wjg.v31.i7.100044

[3] Peleteiro B, Bastos A, Ferro A, Lunet N. Prevalence of *Helicobacter pylori* infection worldwide: A systematic review of studies with national coverage. Digestive Diseases and Sciences. 2014;**59**:1698-1709. DOI: 10.1007/s10620-014-3063-0

[4] Camilo V, Sugiyama T, Touati E. Pathogenesis of *Helicobacter pylori* infection. Helicobacter. 2017;**22**(Suppl):1. DOI: 10.1111/hel.12405

[5] Nishizawa T. Dual therapy for third-line *Helicobacter pylori* eradication and urea breath test prediction. World Journal of Gastroenterology. 2012;**18**:2735. DOI: 10.3748/wjg.v18.i21.2735

[6] Toyoshima O, Nishizawa T, Koike K. Endoscopic Kyoto classification of *Helicobacter pylori* infection and gastric cancer risk diagnosis. World Journal of Gastroenterology. 2020;**26**:466-477. DOI: 10.3748/wjg.v26.i5.466

[7] Toyoshima O, Nishizawa T, Arita M, Kataoka Y, Sakitani K, Yoshida S, et al. *Helicobacter pylori* infection in subjects negative for high titer serum antibody. World Journal of Gastroenterology. 2018;**24**:1419-1428. DOI: 10.3748/wjg.v24.i13.1419

[8] Yoshii S, Mabe K, Watano K, Ohno M, Matsumoto M, Ono S, et al. Validity of endoscopic features for the diagnosis of *Helicobacter pylori* infection status based on the Kyoto classification of gastritis. Digestive Endoscopy. 2020;**32**:74-83. DOI: 10.1111/den.13486

[9] Garcés-Durán R, García-Rodríguez A, Córdova H, Cuatrecasas M, Ginès À, González-Suárez B, et al. Association between a regular arrangement of collecting venules and absence of *Helicobacter pylori* infection in a European population. Gastrointestinal Endoscopy. 2019;**90**:461-466. DOI: 10.1016/j.gie.2019.05.027

[10] Lash JG, Genta RM. Adherence to the Sydney system guidelines increases the detection of *Helicobacter gastritis* and intestinal metaplasia in 400 738 sets of gastric biopsies. Alimentary Pharmacology & Therapeutics. 2013;**38**:424-431. DOI: 10.1111/apt.12383

[11] Rotimi O, Cairns A, Gray S, Moayyedi P, Dixon MF. Histological identification of *Helicobacter pylori*: Comparison of staining methods. Journal of Clinical Pathology. 2000;**53**:756-759. DOI: 10.1136/jcp.53.10.756

[12] Batts KP, Ketover S, Kakar S, Krasinskas AM, Mitchell KA, Wilcox R, et al. Appropriate use of special stains for identifying *Helicobacter pylori*: Recommendations from the Rodger C. Haggitt Gastrointestinal Pathology Society. The American Journal of Surgical Pathology. 2013;**37**:e12-e22. DOI: 10.1097/PAS.0000000000000097

[13] Malfertheiner P, Megraud F, O'Morain CA, Gisbert JP, Kuipers EJ, Axon AT, et al. Management of *Helicobacter pylori* infection—The

Maastricht V/Florence Consensus Report. Gut. 2016;**66**:6-30. DOI: 10.1136/gutjnl-2016-312288

[14] Chey WD, Wong BCY. American College of Gastroenterology guideline on the management of *Helicobacter pylori* infection. The American Journal of Gastroenterology. 2007;**102**:1808-1825. DOI: 10.1111/j.1572-0241.2007.01393.x

[15] Vaira D, Vakil N, Gatta L, Ricci C, Perna F, Saracino I, et al. Accuracy of a new ultrafast rapid urease test to diagnose *Helicobacter pylori* infection in 1000 consecutive dyspeptic patients. Alimentary Pharmacology & Therapeutics. 2010;**31**:331-338. DOI: 10.1111/j.1365-2036.2009.04196.x

[16] Hsu W. Dual specimens increase the diagnostic accuracy and reduce the reaction duration of rapid urease test. World Journal of Gastroenterology. 2010;**16**:2926. DOI: 10.3748/wjg.v16.i23.2926

[17] Moon SW, Kim TH, Kim HS, Ju J, Ahn YJ, Jang HJ, et al. United rapid urease test is superior than separate test in detecting *Helicobacter pylori* at the gastric antrum and body specimens. Clinical Endoscopy. 2012;**45**:392. DOI: 10.5946/ce.2012.45.4.392

[18] Lerang F, Moum B, Mowinckel P, Haug JB, Ragnhildstveit E, Berge T, et al. Accuracy of seven different tests for the diagnosis of *Helicobacter pylori* infection and the impact of H2-receptor antagonists on test results. Scandinavian Journal of Gastroenterology. 1998;**33**:364-369. DOI: 10.1080/00365529850170982

[19] Gisbert JP, Abraira V. Accuracy of *Helicobacter pylori* diagnostic tests in patients with bleeding peptic ulcer: A systematic review and meta-analysis. The American Journal of Gastroenterology. 2006;**101**:848-863. DOI: 10.1111/j.1572-0241.2006.00528.x

[20] Leszczyńska K, Namiot A, Namiot Z, Leszczyńska JK, Jakoniuk P, Chilewicz M, et al. Patient factors affecting culture of *Helicobacter pylori* isolated from gastric mucosal specimens. Advances in Medical Sciences. 2010;**55**:161-166. DOI: 10.2478/v10039-010-0028-1

[21] Mégraud F, Lehours P. *Helicobacter pylori* detection and antimicrobial susceptibility testing. Clinical Microbiology Reviews. 2007;**20**:280-322. DOI: 10.1128/CMR.00033-06

[22] Ndip RN, MacKay WG, Farthing MJ, Weaver LT. Culturing *Helicobacter pylori* from clinical specimens: Review of microbiologic methods. Journal of Pediatric Gastroenterology and Nutrition. 2003;**36**:616-622. DOI: 10.1097/00005176-200305000-00005

[23] Ferwana M. Accuracy of urea breath test in *Helicobacter pylori* infection: Meta-analysis. World Journal of Gastroenterology. 2015;**21**:1305. DOI: 10.3748/wjg.v21.i4.1305

[24] Gisbert JP, Calvet X. *Helicobacter pylori* "test-and-treat" strategy for management of Dyspepsia: A comprehensive review. Clinical and Translational Gastroenterology. 2013;**4**:e32. DOI: 10.1038/ctg.2013.3

[25] Guarner J, Kalach N, Elitsur Y, Koletzko S. *Helicobacter pylori* diagnostic tests in children: Review of the literature from 1999 to 2009. European Journal of Pediatrics. 2010;**169**:15-25. DOI: 10.1007/s00431-009-1033-x

[26] McColl KE. Clinical practice. *Helicobacter pylori* infection. The New England Journal of Medicine.

2010;**362**:1597-1604. DOI: 10.1056/NEJMcp1001110

[27] Velayos B, Fernández-Salazar L, Pons-Renedo F, Muñoz MF, Almaraz A, Aller R, et al. Accuracy of urea breath test performed immediately after emergency endoscopy in peptic ulcer bleeding. Digestive Diseases and Sciences. 2012;**57**:1880-1886. DOI: 10.1007/s10620-012-2096-5

[28] Mana F, Franken PR, Ham HR, Urbain D. Cut-off point, timing and pitfalls of the ^{13}C-urea breath test as measured by infrared spectrometry. Digestive and Liver Disease. 2001;**33**:30-35. DOI: 10.1016/s1590-8658(01)80132-8

[29] Gisbert JP, de la Morena F, Abraira V. Accuracy of monoclonal stool antigen test for the diagnosis of *H. pylori* infection: A systematic review and meta-analysis. The American Journal of Gastroenterology. 2006;**101**:1921-1930

[30] Deguchi R, Matsushima M, Suzuki T, Mine T, Fukuda R, Nishina M, et al. Comparison of a monoclonal with a polyclonal antibody-based enzyme immunoassay stool test in diagnosing *Helicobacter pylori* infection after eradication therapy. Journal of Gastroenterology. 2009;**44**:713-716. DOI: 10.1007/s00535-009-0069-z

[31] Calvet X, Lario S, Ramirez-Lazaro MJ, Montserrat A, Quesada M, Reeves L, et al. Accuracy of monoclonal stool tests for determining cure of *Helicobacter pylori* infection after treatment. Helicobacter. 2010;**15**:201-205. DOI: 10.1111/j.1523-5378.2010.00757.x

[32] Queiroz DMM, Saito M, Rocha GA, Rocha AMC, Melo FF, Checkley W, et al. *Helicobacter pylori* infection in infants and toddlers in South America: Concordance between [^{13}C]urea breath test and monoclonal *H. pylori* stool antigen test. Journal of Clinical Microbiology. 2013;**51**:3735-3740. DOI: 10.1128/JCM.01752-13

[33] Zhou X, Su J, Xu G, Zhang G. Accuracy of stool antigen test for the diagnosis of *Helicobacter pylori* infection in children: A meta-analysis. Clinics and Research in Hepatology and Gastroenterology. 2014;**38**:629-638. DOI: 10.1016/j.clinre.2014.02.001

[34] Demirturk L, Yazgan Y, Tarcin O, Ozel M, Diler M, Oncul O, et al. Does N-acetyl cystein affect the sensitivity and specificity of *Helicobacter pylori* stool antigen test? Helicobacter. 2003;**8**:120-123. DOI: 10.1046/j.1523-5378.2003.00132.x

[35] Shimoyama T. Stool antigen tests for the management of *Helicobacter pylori* infection. World Journal of Gastroenterology. 2013;**19**:8188. DOI: 10.3748/wjg.v19.i45.8188

[36] Miki K. Gastric cancer screening by combined assay for serum anti-*Helicobacter pylori* IgG antibody and serum pepsinogen levels—"ABC method". Proceedings of the Japan Academy. Series B, Physical and Biological Sciences. 2011;**87**:405-414. DOI: 10.2183/pjab.87.405

[37] Takahashi-Kanemitsu A, Knight CT, Hatakeyama M. Molecular anatomy and pathogenic actions of *Helicobacter pylori* CagA that underpin gastric carcinogenesis. Cellular & Molecular Immunology. 2020;**17**:50-63. DOI: 10.1038/s41423-019-0339-5

[38] Li Q, Liu J, Gong Y, Yuan Y. Serum VacA antibody is associated with risks of peptic ulcer and gastric cancer: A meta-analysis. Microbial Pathogenesis. 2016;**99**:220-228. DOI: 10.1016/j.micpath.2016.08.030

[39] El HF, Wang T, Ndifor VM, Jin G. Association between *Helicobacter pylori*

antibodies determined by multiplex serology and gastric cancer risk: A meta-analysis. Helicobacter. 2022;**27**:e12881. DOI: 10.1111/hel.12881

[40] Marchildon PA, Sugiyama T, Fukuda Y, Peacock JS, Asaka M, Shimoyama T, et al. Evaluation of the effects of strain-specific antigen variation on the accuracy of serologic diagnosis of *Helicobacter pylori* infection. Journal of Clinical Microbiology. 2003;**41**:1480-1485. DOI: 10.1128/JCM.41.4.1480-1485.2003

[41] Kabir S. Detection of *Helicobacter pylori* DNA in feces and saliva by polymerase chain reaction: A review. Helicobacter. 2004;**9**:115-123. DOI: 10.1111/j.1083-4389.2004.00207.x

[42] Šeligová B, Lukáč Ľ, Bábelová M, Vávrová S, Sulo P. Diagnostic reliability of nested PCR depends on the primer design and threshold abundance of *Helicobacter pylori* in biopsy, stool, and saliva samples. Helicobacter. 2020;**25**:e12680. DOI: 10.1111/hel.12680

[43] Qiu E, Li Z, Han S. Methods for detection of *Helicobacter pylori* from stool sample: Current options and developments. Brazilian Journal of Microbiology. 2021;**52**:2057-2062. DOI: 10.1007/s42770-021-00589-x

[44] Singh V, Mishra S, Rao GRK, Jain AK, Dixit VK, Gulati AK, et al. Evaluation of nested PCR in detection of *Helicobacter pylori* targeting a highly conserved gene: HSP60. Helicobacter. 2008;**13**:30-34. DOI: 10.1111/j.1523-5378.2008.00573.x

[45] Mishra S, Singh V, Rao GRK, Dixit VK, Gulati AK, Nath G. Prevalence of *Helicobacter pylori* in asymptomatic subjects—A nested PCR based study. Infection, Genetics and Evolution. 2008;**8**:815-819. DOI: 10.1016/j.meegid.2008.08.001

[46] Patel SK. Diagnosis of *Helicobacter pylori*: What should be the gold standard? World Journal of Gastroenterology. 2014;**20**:12847. DOI: 10.3748/wjg.v20.i36.12847

[47] Clayton C, Kleanthous K, Tabaqchali S. Detection and identification of *Helicobacter pylori* by the polymerase chain reaction. Journal of Clinical Pathology. 1991;**44**:515-516. DOI: 10.1136/jcp.44.6.515

[48] Maeda S, Yoshida H, Ogura K, Kanai F, Shiratori Y, Omata M. *Helicobacter pylori* specific nested PCR assay for the detection of 23S rRNA mutation associated with clarithromycin resistance. Gut. 1998;**43**:317-321. DOI: 10.1136/gut.43.3.317

[49] Corless CE, Guiver M, Borrow R, Edwards-Jones V, Kaczmarski EB, Fox AJ. Contamination and sensitivity issues with a real-time universal 16S rRNA PCR. Journal of Clinical Microbiology. 2000;**38**:1747-1752. DOI: 10.1128/JCM.38.5.1747-1752.2000

[50] Demiray Gürbüz E, Yılmaz Ö, Olivares AZ, Gönen C, Sarıoğlu S, Soytürk M, et al. Rapid identification of *Helicobacter pylori* and assessment of clarithromycin susceptibility from clinical specimens using FISH. The Journal of Pathology. Clinical Research. 2017;**3**:29-37. DOI: 10.1002/cjp2.57

[51] Morris JM, Reasonover AL, Bruce MG, Bruden DL, McMahon BJ, Sacco FD, et al. Evaluation of seaFAST, a rapid fluorescent in situ hybridization test, for detection of *Helicobacter pylori* and resistance to clarithromycin in paraffin-embedded biopsy sections. Journal of Clinical Microbiology. 2005;**43**:3494-3496. DOI: 10.1128/JCM.43.7.3494-3496.2005

[52] Vega AE, Alarcón T, Domingo D, López-Brea M. Detection of

clarithromycin-resistant *Helicobacter pylori* in frozen gastric biopsies from pediatric patients by a commercially available fluorescent in situ hybridization. Diagnostic Microbiology and Infectious Disease. 2007;**59**:421-423. DOI: 10.1016/j.diagmicrobio.2007.06.020

[53] Megraud F. H pylori antibiotic resistance: Prevalence, importance, and advances in testing. Gut. 2004;**53**:1374-1384. DOI: 10.1136/gut.2003.022111

[54] Cerqueira L, Fernandes RM, Ferreira RM, Carneiro F, Dinis-Ribeiro M, Figueiredo C, et al. PNA-FISH as a new diagnostic method for the determination of clarithromycin resistance of *Helicobacter pylori*. BMC Microbiology. 2011;**11**:101. DOI: 10.1186/1471-2180-11-101

[55] Saracino IM, Pavoni M, Zullo A, Fiorini G, Lazzarotto T, Borghi C, et al. Next generation sequencing for the prediction of the antibiotic resistance in *Helicobacter pylori*: A literature review. Antibiotics (Basel). 2021;**10**:437. DOI: 10.3390/antibiotics10040437

[56] Kumar KR, Cowley MJ, Davis RL. Next-generation sequencing and emerging technologies. Seminars in Thrombosis and Hemostasis. 2019;**45**:661-673. DOI: 10.1055/s-0039-1688446

[57] Engstrand L. How will next-generation sequencing contribute to the knowledge concerning *Helicobacter pylori*? Clinical Microbiology and Infection. 2009;**15**:823-828. DOI: 10.1111/j.1469-0691.2009.02962.x

[58] Lauener F, Imkamp F, Lehours P, Buissonnière A, Benejat L, Zbinden R, et al. Genetic determinants and prediction of antibiotic resistance phenotypes in *Helicobacter pylori*. Journal of Clinical Medicine. 2019;**8**:53. DOI: 10.3390/jcm8010053

[59] Gillet L, Benejat L, Jehanne Q, Maunet P, Perreau C, Ducournau A, et al. Resistome and virulome determination in *Helicobacter pylori* using next-generation sequencing with target-enrichment technology. Microbiology Spectrum. 2025;**13**:e329824. DOI: 10.1128/spectrum.03298-24

[60] Thorell K, Bengtsson-Palme J, Liu OH, Palacios GR, Nookaew I, Rabeneck L, et al. In vivo analysis of the viable microbiota and *Helicobacter pylori* transcriptome in gastric infection and early stages of carcinogenesis. Infection and Immunity. 2017;**85**:e00031-17. DOI: 10.1128/IAI.00031-17

[61] Zhao X, Zhang H, Li D, Zhou J, Chen Y, Sun Y, et al. Whole-genome sequencing reveals origin and evolution of influenza A(H1N1)pdm09 viruses in Lincang, China, from 2014 to 2018. PLoS ONE. 2020;**15**:e234869. DOI: 10.1371/journal.pone.0234869

[62] Humphreys H, Coleman DC. Contribution of whole-genome sequencing to understanding of the epidemiology and control of meticillin-resistant Staphylococcus aureus. The Journal of Hospital Infection. 2019;**102**:189-199. DOI: 10.1016/j.jhin.2019.01.025

[63] Pohl D, Keller PM, Bordier V, Wagner K. Review of current diagnostic methods and advances in *Helicobacter pylori* diagnostics in the era of next generation sequencing. World Journal of Gastroenterology. 2019;**25**:4629-4660. DOI: 10.3748/wjg.v25.i32.4629

[64] Kaminski MM, Abudayyeh OO, Gootenberg JS, Zhang F, Collins JJ. CRISPR-based diagnostics. Nature

Biomedical Engineering. 2021;**5**:643-656. DOI: 10.1038/s41551-021-00760-7

[65] Qiu E, Jin S, Xiao Z, Chen Q, Wang Q, Liu H, et al. CRISPR-based detection of *Helicobacter pylori* in stool samples. Helicobacter. 2021;**26**:e12828. DOI: 10.1111/hel.12828

[66] Dai B, Xiang A, Qu D, Chen G, Wang L, Wang W, et al. Rapid and sensitive assay of *Helicobacter pylori* with one-tube RPA-CRISPR/Cas12 by portable array detector for visible analysis of thermostatic nucleic acid amplification. Frontiers in Microbiology. 2022;**13**:858247. DOI: 10.3389/fmicb.2022.858247

[67] Wang Y, Liu L, Liu X, Wu K, Zhu X, Ma L, et al. An ultrasensitive PCR-based CRISPR-Cas13a method for the detection of *Helicobacter pylori*. Journal of Personalized Medicine. 2022;**12**:2082. DOI: 10.3390/jpm12122082

[68] Liu H, Wang J, Hu X, Tang X, Zhang C. A rapid and high-throughput *Helicobacter pylori* RPA-CRISPR/Cas12a-based nucleic acid detection system. Clinica Chimica Acta. 2023;**540**:117201. DOI: 10.1016/j.cca.2022.12.013

[69] Zhu R, Jiang H, Li C, Li Y, Peng M, Wang J, et al. CRISPR/Cas9-based point-of-care lateral flow biosensor with improved performance for rapid and robust detection of *Mycoplasma pneumonia*. Analytica Chimica Acta. 2023;**1257**:341175. DOI: 10.1016/j.aca.2023.341175

[70] Yan K, Wang X, Han Y, Tian Y, Niu M, Dong X, et al. Simultaneous detection of *Helicobacter pylori* and clarithromycin resistance mutations using RAA-CRISPR/Cas13a assay. Infection and Drug Resistance. 2024;**17**:3001-3010. DOI: 10.2147/IDR.S462963

[71] Nolan T, Hands RE, Ogunkolade W, Bustin SA. SPUD: A quantitative PCR assay for the detection of inhibitors in nucleic acid preparations. Analytical Biochemistry. 2006;**351**:308-310. DOI: 10.1016/j.ab.2006.01.051

[72] Gupta D, Bhattacharjee O, Mandal D, Sen MK, Dey D, Dasgupta A, et al. CRISPR-Cas9 system: A new-fangled dawn in gene editing. Life Sciences. 2019;**232**:116636. DOI: 10.1016/j.lfs.2019.116636

[73] Salama N, Guillemin K, McDaniel TK, Sherlock G, Tompkins L, Falkow S. A whole-genome microarray reveals genetic diversity among *Helicobacter pylori* strains. Proceedings of the National Academy of Sciences of the United States of America. 2000;**97**:14668-14673. DOI: 10.1073/pnas.97.26.14668

[74] Xuan S, Zhou Y, Shao B, Cui Y, Li J, Yin H, et al. Enzymic colorimetry-based DNA chip: A rapid and accurate assay for detecting mutations for clarithromycin resistance in the 23S rRNA gene of *Helicobacter pylori*. Journal of Medical Microbiology. 2009;**58**:1443-1448. DOI: 10.1099/jmm.0.010785-0

[75] Chen S, Li Y, Yu C. Oligonucleotide microarray: A new rapid method for screening the 23S rRNA gene of *Helicobacter pylori* for single nucleotide polymorphisms associated with clarithromycin resistance. Journal of Gastroenterology and Hepatology. 2008;**23**:126-131. DOI: 10.1111/j.1440-1746.2007.04900.x

[76] Yin G, Bie S, Gu H, Shu X, Zheng W, Peng K, et al. Application of gene chip technology in the diagnostic and drug resistance detection of *Helicobacter pylori* in children. Journal of Gastroenterology and Hepatology. 2020;**35**:1331-1339. DOI: 10.1111/jgh.14980

[77] Xing JZ, Clarke C, Zhu L, Gabos S. Development of a microelectronic chip array for high-throughput genotyping of Helicobacter species and screening for antimicrobial resistance. Journal of Biomolecular Screening. 2005;**10**:235-245. DOI: 10.1177/1087057104273781

[78] Halperin A, Buhot A, Zhulina EB. Sensitivity, specificity, and the hybridization isotherms of DNA chips. Biophysical Journal. 2004;**86**:718-730. DOI: 10.1016/S0006-3495(04)74150-8

[79] Xuan SH, Wu LP, Zhou YG, Xiao MB. Detection of clarithromycin-resistant *Helicobacter pylori* in clinical specimens by molecular methods: A review. Journal of Global Antimicrobial Resistance. 2016;**4**:35-41. DOI: 10.1016/j.jgar.2016.01.002

[80] Tsuchida S, Umemura H, Nakayama T. Current status of matrix-assisted laser desorption/ionization–time-of-flight mass spectrometry (MALDI-TOF MS) in clinical diagnostic microbiology. Molecules. 2020;**25**:4775. DOI: 10.3390/molecules25204775

[81] Berlamont H, De Witte C, De Bruyckere S, Fox JG, Backert S, Smet A, et al. Differentiation of gastric Helicobacter species using MALDI-TOF mass spectrometry. Pathogens. 2021;**10**:366. DOI: 10.3390/pathogens10030366

[82] Taniguchi T, Sekiya A, Higa M, Saeki Y, Umeki K, Okayama A, et al. Rapid identification and subtyping of *Helicobacter cinaedi* strains by intact-cell mass spectrometry profiling with the use of matrix-assisted laser desorption ionization-time of flight mass spectrometry. Journal of Clinical Microbiology. 2014;**52**:95-102. DOI: 10.1128/JCM.01798-13

[83] Cardos AI, Maghiar A, Zaha DC, Pop O, Fritea L, Miere Groza F, et al. Evolution of diagnostic methods for *Helicobacter pylori* infections: From traditional tests to high technology, advanced sensitivity and discrimination tools. Diagnostics (Basel). 2022;**12**:508. DOI: 10.3390/diagnostics12020508

[84] Wieser A, Schneider L, Jung J, Schubert S. MALDI-TOF MS in microbiological diagnostics-identification of microorganisms and beyond (mini review). Applied Microbiology and Biotechnology. 2012;**93**:965-974. DOI: 10.1007/s00253-011-3783-4

[85] Chen JHK, Ho P, Kwan GSW, She KKK, Siu GKH, Cheng VCC, et al. Direct bacterial identification in positive blood cultures by use of two commercial matrix-assisted laser desorption ionization–time of flight mass spectrometry systems. Journal of Clinical Microbiology. 2013;**51**:1733-1739. DOI: 10.1128/JCM.03259-12

[86] Kitagawa K, Shigemura K, Onuma KI, Nishida M, Fujiwara M, Kobayashi S, et al. Improved bacterial identification directly from urine samples with matrix-assisted laser desorption/ionization time-of-flight mass spectrometry. Journal of Clinical Laboratory Analysis. 2018;**32**:e22301. DOI: 10.1002/jcla.22301

[87] Oviano M, Rodriguez-Sanchez B, Gomara M, Alcala L, Zvezdanova E, Ruiz A, et al. Direct identification of clinical pathogens from liquid culture media by MALDI-TOF MS analysis. Clinical Microbiology and Infection. 2018;**24**:624-629. DOI: 10.1016/j.cmi.2017.09.010

[88] Matos R, De Witte C, Smet A, Berlamont H, De Bruyckere S, Amorim I, et al. Antimicrobial susceptibility pattern of *Helicobacter heilmannii* and *Helicobacter ailurogastricus*

isolates. Microorganisms. 2020;**8**:957. DOI: 10.3390/microorganisms8060957

[89] Singhal N, Kumar M, Kanaujia PK, Virdi JS. MALDI-TOF mass spectrometry: An emerging technology for microbial identification and diagnosis. Frontiers in Microbiology. 2015;**6**:00791. DOI: 10.3389/fmicb.2015.00791

[90] Chao C, Wang C, Che Y, Kao C, Wu J, Lee G. An integrated microfluidic system for diagnosis of the resistance of *Helicobacter pylori* to quinolone-based antibiotics. Biosensors & Bioelectronics. 2016;**78**:281-289. DOI: 10.1016/j.bios.2015.11.046

[91] Filomena A, Guenther A, Planatscher H, Topin F, She J, Formichella L, et al. Performance of a multiplex serological *Helicobacter pylori* assay on a novel microfluidic assay platform. Proteomes. 2017;**5**:24. DOI: 10.3390/proteomes5040024

[92] Pereira SV, Messina GA, Raba J. Integrated microfluidic magnetic immunosensor for quantification of human serum IgG antibodies to *Helicobacter pylori*. Journal of Chromatography B. 2010;**878**:253-257. DOI: 10.1016/j.jchromb.2009.05.007

[93] Zhao Y, Chen F, Li Q, Wang L, Fan C. Isothermal amplification of nucleic acids. Chemical Reviews. 2015;**115**:12491-12545. DOI: 10.1021/acs.chemrev.5b00428

[94] Liu J, Fu R, Zhang S, Hou J, Ma H, Hu S, et al. Rapid and multi-target genotyping of *Helicobacter pylori* with digital microfluidics. Biosensors & Bioelectronics. 2024;**256**:116282. DOI: 10.1016/j.bios.2024.116282

[95] Fabini E, Zambelli B, Mazzei L, Ciurli S, Bertucci C. Surface plasmon resonance and isothermal titration calorimetry to monitor the Ni(II)-dependent binding of *Helicobacter pylori* NikR to DNA. Analytical and Bioanalytical Chemistry. 2016;**408**:7971-7980. DOI: 10.1007/s00216-016-9894-0

[96] Dubey AK, Kumar Gupta V, Kujawska M, Orive G, Kim N, Li C, et al. Exploring nano-enabled CRISPR-Cas-powered strategies for efficient diagnostics and treatment of infectious diseases. Journal of Nanostructure in Chemistry. 2022;**12**:833-864. DOI: 10.1007/s40097-022-00472-7

[97] Tsuda M, Watanabe Y, Oikawa R, Watanabe R, Higashino M, Kubo K, et al. Clinical evaluation of a novel molecular diagnosis kit for detecting *Helicobacter pylori* and clarithromycin-resistant using intragastric fluid. Helicobacter. 2022;**27**:e12933. DOI: 10.1111/hel.12933

[98] Schulz C, Kalali B, Link A, Gerhard M, Malfertheiner P. New rapid *Helicobacter pylori* blood test based on dual detection of FliD and CagA antibodies for on-site testing. Clinical Gastroenterology and Hepatology. 2023;**21**:229-231. DOI: 10.1016/j.cgh.2021.11.008

[99] Pang X, Fu Q, Yang Y, Zhou C, Feng S, Gong K, et al. A low-voltage alternant direct current electroporation chip for ultrafast releasing the genome DNA of *Helicobacter pylori* bacterium. Mikrochimica Acta. 2024;**191**:116. DOI: 10.1007/s00604-024-06187-6

[100] Chen C, Liou J, Lee Y, Hong T, El-Omar EM, Wu M. The interplay between *Helicobacter pylori* and gastrointestinal microbiota. Gut Microbes. 2021;**13**:1-22. DOI: 10.1080/19490976.2021.1909459

[101] Felley C, Michetti P. Probiotics and *Helicobacter pylori*. Best Practice & Research Clinical Gastroenterology. 2003;**17**:785-791. DOI: 10.1016/s1521-6918(03)00070-2

[102] Nomura R, Kadota T, Ogaya Y, Matayoshi S, Iwashita N, Okawa R, et al. Contribution of Streptococcus mutans to *Helicobacter pylori* colonisation in oral cavity and gastric tissue. Scientific Reports. 2020;**10**:12540. DOI: 10.1038/s41598-020-69368-2

[103] Peng L, Guo Y, Gerhard M, Gao J, Liu Z, Mejías-Luque R, et al. Metabolite alterations and interactions with microbiota in *Helicobacter pylori*-associated gastric lesions. Microbiology Spectrum. 2023;**11**:e0534722. DOI: 10.1128/spectrum.05347-22

[104] Bakhti SZ, Latifi-Navid S. Oral microbiota and *Helicobacter pylori* in gastric carcinogenesis: What do we know and where next? BMC Microbiology. 2021;**21**:71. DOI: 10.1186/s12866-021-02130-4

[105] Dai D, Yang Y, Yu J, Dang T, Qin W, Teng L, et al. Interactions between gastric microbiota and metabolites in gastric cancer. Cell Death & Disease. 2021;**12**:1104. DOI: 10.1038/s41419-021-04396-y

[106] Abbondio M, Tanca A, De Diego L, Sau R, Bibbò S, Pes GM, et al. Metaproteomic assessment of gut microbial and host functional perturbations in *Helicobacter pylori*-infected patients subjected to an antimicrobial protocol. Gut Microbes. 2023;**15**:2291170. DOI: 10.1080/19490976.2023.2291170

[107] Liatsos C, Papaefthymiou A, Kyriakos N, Galanopoulos M, Doulberis M, Giakoumis M, et al. *Helicobacter pylori*, gastric microbiota and gastric cancer relationship: Unrolling the tangle. World Journal of Gastrointestinal Oncology. 2022;**14**:959-972. DOI: 10.4251/wjgo.v14.i5.959

[108] Zou P, Zhu J, Zhao Z, Mei H, Zhao J, Sun W, et al. Development and application of an artificial intelligence-assisted endoscopy system for diagnosis of *Helicobacter pylori* infection: A multicenter randomized controlled study. BMC Gastroenterology. 2024;**24**:335. DOI: 10.1186/s12876-024-03389-3

[109] Shen Y, Chen A, Zhang X, Zhong X, Ma A, Wang J, et al. Real-time evaluation of *Helicobacter pylori* infection by convolution neural network during white-light endoscopy: A prospective, multicenter study (with video). Clinical and Translational Gastroenterology. 2023;**14**:e643. DOI: 10.14309/ctg.0000000000000643

[110] Martin DR, Hanson JA, Gullapalli RR, Schultz FA, Sethi A, Clark DP. A deep learning convolutional neural network can recognize common patterns of injury in gastric pathology. Archives of Pathology & Laboratory Medicine. 2020;**144**:370-378. DOI: 10.5858/arpa.2019-0004-OA

[111] Klein S, Gildenblat J, Ihle MA, Merkelbach-Bruse S, Noh K, Peifer M, et al. Deep learning for sensitive detection of *Helicobacter pylori* in gastric biopsies. BMC Gastroenterology. 2020;**20**:417. DOI: 10.1186/s12876-020-01494-7

[112] Liscia DS, D'Andrea M, Biletta E, Bellis D, Demo K, Ferrero F, et al. Use of digital pathology and artificial intelligence for the diagnosis of *Helicobacter pylori* in gastric biopsies. Pathologica. 2022;**114**:295-303. DOI: 10.32074/1591-951X-751

[113] Qin Q, Wang K, Yang J, Xu H, Cao B, Wo Y, et al. Algorithms for immunochromatographic assay: Review and impact on future application. The Analyst. 2019;**144**:5659-5676. DOI: 10.1039/c9an00964g

Chapter 4

Understanding Antibiotic Resistance Mechanisms in *H. pylori* and Its Clinical Implications

Kareem Ibraheem, Osama Hroub, Abdalrahman N. Herbawi and Majed Dwaik

Abstract

Helicobacter pylori, infecting half of the global population, is a major cause of gastroduodenal disorders, including peptic ulcers, gastric cancer, and mucosa-associated lymphoid tissue lymphoma. Resistance to antibiotics, driven by genetic mutations (e.g., 23 s rRNA, gyrA) and efflux pump activation, has severely compromised eradication therapies. Raising resistance to clarithromycin, metronidazole, and levofloxacin reduces the effectiveness of first-line treatments such as triple therapy, requiring alternatives such as quadruple bismuth therapy, sequential regimes, and susceptibility-guided approaches. Socioeconomic factors, improper use of antibiotics, and low treatment adherence further exacerbate resistance. Clinically, resistance increases treatment failures, recurrence of complications, and cancer risk. Strategies for mitigating resistance include global vigilance, probiotics as adjuncts, and personalized therapies guided by molecular diagnoses. The confrontation of these challenges requires updated guidelines, regional monitoring of resistance, and public health interventions to optimize eradication and reduce the load of diseases.

Keywords: antibiotic resistance, eradication failure, genetic mutations, *Helicobacter pylori* eradication, *Helicobacter pylori* resistance, clinical implications

1. Introduction

Bacterial infection of *Helicobacter pylori* (*H. pylori*) affects almost half of the global population, with prevalence rates reaching up to 70% in developing countries compared to 40% in developed ones [1]. Oral and fecal transmission are primary propagation modes, usually linked to bad sanitation, contaminated drinking water, and overcrowded living conditions. Although many carriers remain thus, *H. pylori* is a major cause of chronic gastritis, peptic ulcer, gastric cancer, and lymphoid lymphoma associated with mucosa [2, 3]. In addition, its persistence in the stomach leads to inflammation, immune dropout, and resistance to conventional treatments, complicating disease management efforts and eradication.

Eventually, the micro-organism affects the protective barrier of the mucosa, reasons inflammatory responses within the stomach mucosa, and raises acid generation, therefore causing mucosal harm and ulcers. Infection rates are extraordinarily stimulated by socioeconomic degree, hygienic practices, and consuming conduct; so, those troubles constitute a first-rate public health problem [4]. Apart from peptic ulcers, *H. Pylori* infection is a genuine cause of stomach adenocarcinoma, the third maximum regular purpose of most cancer mortality globally. Chronic infection opens the course for malignant transformation through inflicting dysplasia, intestinal metaplasia, and atrophic gastritis [5].

Furthermore, connected to mucosa-associated lymphoid tissue (MALT) lymphoma, an unprecedented stomach tumor that could get better after bacterial eradication [6] is also their involvement. Reducing the weight of *H. Pylori*-related diseases depends severely on suitable screening, early eradication, right treatment, and surveillance for resistance, given such major medical effects.

2. *H. pylori* eradication is significant in reducing the burden of disease

2.1 The importance of *H. pylori* eradication in gastrointestinal disease prevention and treatment

Several gastrointestinal diseases cannot be prevented or treated without eradicating *H. pylori*. Since reinfection is infrequent in many geographic areas among adults, good eradication treatment greatly lowers the chance of peptic ulcer recurrence. Eradication also has a key role in preventing gastric cancer, especially in those who already have precancerous conditions, including intestinal metaplasia and atrophic gastritis [7]. Studies have shown that the treatment of an *H. pylori* infection reduces the incidence of stomach cancer, especially if done before irreversible mucosal changes occur. Early diagnosis and treatment significantly improve outcomes. In addition, lymphoid lymphoma associated with mucosa (MALT) can refer as a result of eradication therapy, reducing the need for more intensive therapies such as chemotherapy or radiation [8]. Successful eradication increases general gastric health and reduces the load of diseases.

2.2 The antibiotic resistance issue and its impact on treatment success rates

The rising resistance of *H. Pylori* to antibiotics is a vital obstacle to eradication therapy, because it results in accelerated treatment failure costs, and prolonged contamination-associated headaches. Conventionally, the first-line triple remedy comprising a proton pump inhibitor (PPI), clarithromycin, and amoxicillin or metronidazole showed excellent efficacy, with eradication prices exceeding 85% [9]. However, because of resistance to clarithromycin exceeding 20% in maximum areas [10], the effectiveness of this routine has dropped to less than 60% in resistant strains. Similarly, resistance to metronidazole and levofloxacin has also confined other remedy alternatives, in particular in areas where there's rampant antibiotic misuse, improper prescriptions, and lack of patient adherence [11]. This, therefore, subjects patients to a couple of tries at remedy, increasing healthcare expenses, aspect results, and the likelihood of further resistance. Failure of the initial eradication remedy not simplest keeps the hazard of recurrent peptic ulcers and dyspepsia but also persists the inflammatory milieu that allows the evolution of gastric cancer [12].

Continuous antibiotic management can alter the gut microbiota, resulting in dysbiosis and likely long-term health outcomes [13].

Because of these boundaries, remedy techniques had been advanced that consist of bismuth quadruple therapy, dual high-dose therapy, and regimens individualized in line with resistance testing [10]. Also, molecular diagnostic technology are getting used increasingly more to become aware of resistance mutations, which allows individualized treatment to beautify healing results [14].

3. Mechanisms and causes of *H. pylori* antibiotic resistance

3.1 Environmental and cultural causes

These trends are in large part fueled by means of the huge misuse of antibiotics, which exerts selective stress on bacterial populations, allowing resistant strains to thrive. For instance, empirical use of clarithromycin-primarily based triple remedy—a routine combining a proton pump inhibitor (PPI), clarithromycin, and amoxicillin or metronidazole—has continued in areas like Europe and East Asia, regardless of clarithromycin resistance exceeding 20–40% [15, 16].

Clarithromycin-based triple regimen remains the first-line in several guidelines, yet Maastricht VI/Florence Reclies Considuits (2022) against its use in the map. Drivers include:

1. Clinical limitations: Endoscopic biopsy and culture are aggressive and expensive, depending on empirical treatment.

2. Guidelines-exercise intervals: Local protocols are behind unanimous updates; for example, Japan recently adopted the recent tailored therapy [17].

3. Economic factor: Sensitivity tests increase the cost, in favor of cheap empirical approaches in resource-limited settings.

This practice has rendered traditional healing procedures useless, with eradication costs losing underneath 60% in excessive-resistance regions [10].

Antibiotic Misuse in *H. Pylori* management is not only a clinical issue, but a systemic failure that requires responsible action. Major priorities include: a global monitoring network to track resistance in real time (e.g., WHO guidelines). Subsidy diagnosis to change empirical therapy in low-resource settings. A public awareness campaign to reduce self-medication and reduce the demand for antibiotics.

Incomplete treatment guides similarly compound the trouble; up to 20% of sufferers discontinue remedy in advance due to aspect effects or socioeconomic obstacles, permitting partly resistant subpopulations to live to tell the tale and propagate [18]. Socioeconomic factors, such as drug costs and restrained healthcare get admission to, disproportionately affect low-income populations, even as low health literacy leads sufferers to stop treatment prematurely once symptoms clear up [19].

Premature discontinuation allows in part resistant bacterial subpopulations to continue to exist, fueling antibiotic resistance, particularly to clarithromycin, which has more and more resistance costs globally, contributing to treatment failure and prolonged infection durations [20].

Socioeconomic interventions, together with subsidized medications, include government or non-governmental organization-funded packages that reduce out-of-pocket charges for antibiotics and PPIs. Community medical examiner applications mitigate access boundaries, even as affected person schooling and digital adherence equipment (e.g., SMS reminders) reinforce compliance with the medication remedy. Education in neighborhood languages, dispelling myths about antibiotics, and improved access for low-income populations through universal health insurance are also essential.

3.2 Genetic causes

Antibiotic resistance in *H. pylori* is mainly from de novo genetic mutations that disrupt the activity of antibiotics by either altering the drug target or inhibiting drug activation within cells (**Table 1**, **Figure 1**) [21].

Macrolides like clarithromycin inhibit protein synthesis by way of binding to the 50S ribosomal subunit, mainly domain V of the 23S rRNA. Resistance in *H. Pylori* typically arises via point mutations inside the 23S rRNA gene, maximum commonly A2143G (adenine to guanine at function 2143) and A2142G, which regulate the ribosome's shape. These mutations disrupt hydrogen bonding and introduce steric quandary, decreasing clarithromycin's affinity with the aid [22]. At the molecular stage, resistance arises through mutations in genes encoding antibiotic goals or drug-activating enzymes. For instance, point mutations in the 23S rRNA gene—mainly A2143G and A2142G—disrupt clarithromycin binding to the bacterial ribosome, accounting for over 90% of macrolide resistance instances [23].

H. Pylori has two 23 s RNA gene copies and resistance requires mutation in both allele (identical), as asymmetric strains can maintain partial sensitivity. This dual-copy requirement complicates resistance development but also explains why resistance rates are correlated with macrolides exposure [24].

Similarly, mutations in the gyrA gene (e.g., N87K, D91G) alter the DNA gyrase enzyme, reducing levofloxacin efficacy by 80% [25, 26]. Cross-resistance from

Antibiotics	Antibiotic resistance mechanism	Associated gene or sequence
Amoxicillin	Mutational change of penicillin-binding protein	*pbp1A, pbp2, pbp3, pbp4*
	Production of beta-lactamase	
	Outer membrane protein mutations causing decreased membrane permeability	*hefC, hopC, hofH*
Clarithromycin	Point mutations in 23S rRNA	23S rRNA
	Increased antibiotic efflux mediated by efflux pump systems	*rpl22, infB*
Levofloxacin	Point mutations in quinolone resistance determination region of DNA gyrase gene	*gyrA, gyrB*
Metronidazole	Mutations causing reduced or abolished nitroreductase activity	*rdxA, frxA*
Tetracycline	Mutations in 16S rRNA	16S rRNA
Rifabutin	Point mutations in rifampicin-resistance determining region of RNA polymerase gene	*rpoB*

Table 1.
Mechanisms of antibiotic resistance in H. pylori.

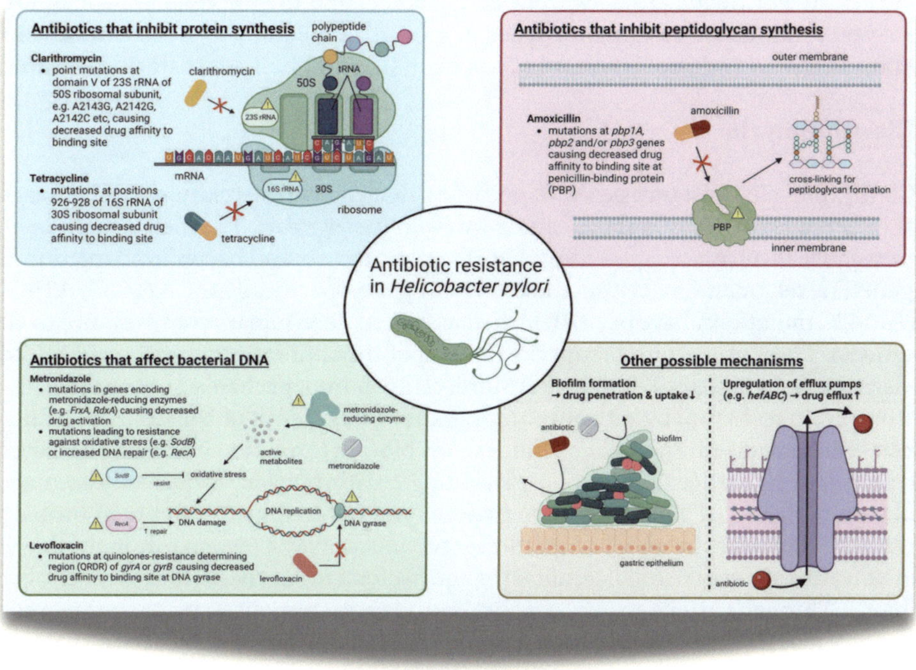

Figure 1.
Mechanisms of resistance to amoxicillin, tetracycline, clarithromycin, metronidazole, levofloxacin, and other mechanisms in Helicobacter pylori.

antibiotics prescribed for unrelated infections, which include fluoroquinolones for urinary tract infections, has also contributed to rising levofloxacin resistance, now exceeding 35% in parts of Europe [27].

Efflux pumps, exemplified by the hefABC system, play a pivotal role in promoting antibiotic resistance by expelling crucial medications such as clarithromycin and metronidazole from bacterial cells. By actively reducing intracellular drug concentrations, these mechanisms significantly diminish the effectiveness of antimicrobial treatments. Unfortunately, the impact of efflux pumps is further compounded by *Helicobacter pylori*'s remarkable genetic adaptability [23]. Leveraging its natural competence and lacking DNA repair systems, *H. pylori* swiftly evolves in response to antimicrobial challenges. This synergistic combination of efflux pumps and genetic plasticity underscores the urgent need for innovative approaches in combating antibiotic resistance within bacterial populations. Stay informed on how these complex factors contribute to the escalating global health crisis and the development of potential solutions [28].

The classification by the World Health Organization (WHO) of clarithromycin-resistant *H. pylori* as a high-priority pathogen underscores the severe and imminent threat it poses to global health. Urging for enhanced surveillance and the development of innovative strategies is therefore imperative to effectively address and contain this escalating concern. The WHO's call for coordinated efforts on an international scale highlights the need for swift and decisive action to combat the growing resistance of *H. pylori* to clarithromycin. By prioritizing this issue and encouraging collaborative measures, the WHO aims to stem the spread of this resistant pathogen and safeguard public health worldwide [29]. Awareness, vigilance, and the implementation of targeted interventions are essential in order to minimize the impact of clarithromycin-resistant *H. pylori* and protect populations from its potentially devastating effects.

3.3 Clarithromycin

Clarithromycin resistance poses a significant challenge in the treatment of various bacterial infections, particularly those caused by *Helicobacter pylori*. The mechanisms behind this resistance involve a complex interplay of genetic factors and bacterial adaptation. At the genetic level, mutations within the 23S rRNA gene, specifically the A2142G, A2143G, and A2142C mutations, have been identified as crucial determinants of resistance to clarithromycin. These mutations disrupt the binding of the antibiotic to the ribosome, leading to a decrease in its efficacy [29]. Furthermore, efflux pump mechanisms play a role in clarithromycin resistance by actively pumping the antibiotic out of bacterial cells, limiting its intracellular concentration [23]. Additionally, biofilm formation has been associated with increased resistance to antibiotics, including clarithromycin. Bacteria encased within biofilms exhibit altered gene expression patterns and reduced susceptibility to antibiotic agents [30]. Moreover, bacterial adaptation mechanisms play a pivotal role in the development of clarithromycin resistance, allowing the bacteria to survive in the presence of the antibiotic. Through various genetic changes and adaptive responses, bacteria can evade the bactericidal effects of clarithromycin and persist in the face of treatment challenges.

3.4 Metronidazole

H. pylori metronidazole resistance represents a significant challenge for effective eradication therapies, contributing to treatment failures and persistent infections. This resistance arises mainly from mutations in genes that encode nitroreductase enzymes such as RDXA gene and FRXA gene, which are critical to activate metronidazole in its cytotoxic form. These mutations impair the activation of the drug, allowing bacteria to avoid its bactericidal effects. In addition, anaerobic stomach conditions increase metronidazole activity, but *H. pylori* may develop adaptive mechanisms to mitigate oxidative stress, further promoting resistance [21]. Globally, resistance rates vary, exceeding 50% in many developing countries, probably due to widespread empirical use of metronidazole for parasitic infections without susceptibility tests, promoting cross-resistance.

On the other hand, regions with stricter antibiotic guidelines report lower rates. Clinically, metronidazole resistance undermines the efficacy of first-line triple therapies (proton pump inhibitor, clarithromycin, and amoxicillin/metronidazole), requiring alternative regimes such as bismuth-based quadruply therapy or fluoroquinolone/rifabutin combinations [31]. The susceptibility test via culture or molecular methods (polymerase chain reaction (PCR) for RDXA/FRXA mutations) is vital for personalized treatment but remains underused in limited-resource configurations. To combat resistance, administration of antibiotics, adherence to therapies combined with adjuvants (e.g., bismuth), and avoidance of metronidazole monotherapy are crucial.

3.5 Levofloxacin

Levofloxacin resistance in *H. Pylori* emerged as a critical barrier to successful eradication, particularly in regions where fluoroquinolones are used in excess for other infections. The resistance is mainly due to mutations in the gyrA gene, which encodes gyrase DNA a load-driven enzyme. Point mutations in the gyrA quinolone resistance region (e.g., in Codons N87 and D91) reduce the affinity of connection to the drug, making the antibiotic ineffective. Positive regulation of the efflux pump can also contribute, although this mechanism is less well characterized. Globally, resistance rates vary widely, exceeding 30% in areas such as Europe, East Asia, and Latin America, driven by the empirical use of levofloxacin for urinary or respiratory infections, which promotes *H. pylori* cross-resistance in cross-resistance [32].

Clinically, levofloxacin resistance compromises second-line therapies, such as levofloxacin-based triple regimens (proton pump inhibitor, amoxicillin, and levofloxacin), forcing reliance on complex alternatives like bismuth quadruple therapy, rifabutin-based protocols, or high-dose dual therapies. Susceptibility testing via molecular methods (PCR for gyrA mutations) or agar dilution is essential for guiding treatment but remains underused in low-resource settings [32].

3.6 Other resistances

Amoxicillin resistance in *H. pylori* is rare but concerning due to the drug's pivotal role in first-line therapies [33]. Clinically, resistance compromises regimens for penicillin-allergic patients, necessitating alternatives like tetracycline- or rifabutin-based therapies. Tetracycline resistance is uncommon but linked to mutations in the 16S rRNA gene, which disrupt the antibiotic's binding to the 30S ribosomal subunit. These mutations are rare due to tetracycline's limited use in modern *H. pylori* regimens, though resistance rates may rise in regions with historical overuse [34]. Rifabutin resistance stems from mutations in the rpoB gene, particularly in the rifampin resistance-determining region (RRDR), such as H540N. These mutations impair rifabutin's binding to RNA polymerase, rendering it ineffective. Cross-resistance with rifampin (used for tuberculosis) is a concern, especially in TB-endemic areas [35].

4. Global trends and epidemiology of resistance

The prevalence of *H. pylori* infection globally is approximately 50%, with rates as high as 80–90% in developing countries and around 35–40% in the United States [36]. Approximately 20% of those infected develop related gastroduodenal disorders during their lifetime. *H. pylori* symptomatic infection treatment regimens usually involve complicated combinations of antimicrobial agents, usually requiring at least 2 weeks of therapy. The most common regimes include triple therapy with two antibiotics, such as metronidazole, amoxicillin, tetracycline, or clarithromycin, combined with a proton pump inhibitor or bismuth [36]. Antimicrobial resistance represents a significant challenge in *H. pylori* treatment, with studies indicating that resistance to multiple agents is predominant. The *H. pylori* antimicrobial resistance monitoring program (HARP) reported that of the 347 clinical isolates collected from December 1998 to 2002, 29.1% exhibited resistance to at least one antimicrobial agent, and 4.8% were resistant to two or more. Resistance to metronidazole was observed in 25.1% of isolates, while 12.9% were resistant to clarithromycin, and 0.9% to amoxicillin [36].

The prevalence of antibiotic resistance in *H. pylori* infections varies significantly across different regions of the world. In Europe and the USA, the resistance to metronidazole is reported to be between 20% and 40%, with a notable exception of higher resistance observed in Northern Italy. In contrast, the Americas and Southeast Asia regions show a lower resistance rate of approximately 10% [16].

A comprehensive evaluation of primary resistance in newly diagnosed *H. pylori* patients indicates that the prevalence of metronidazole resistance is about 38.1% [37]. Furthermore, the resistance rates for other antibiotics are concerning; for instance,

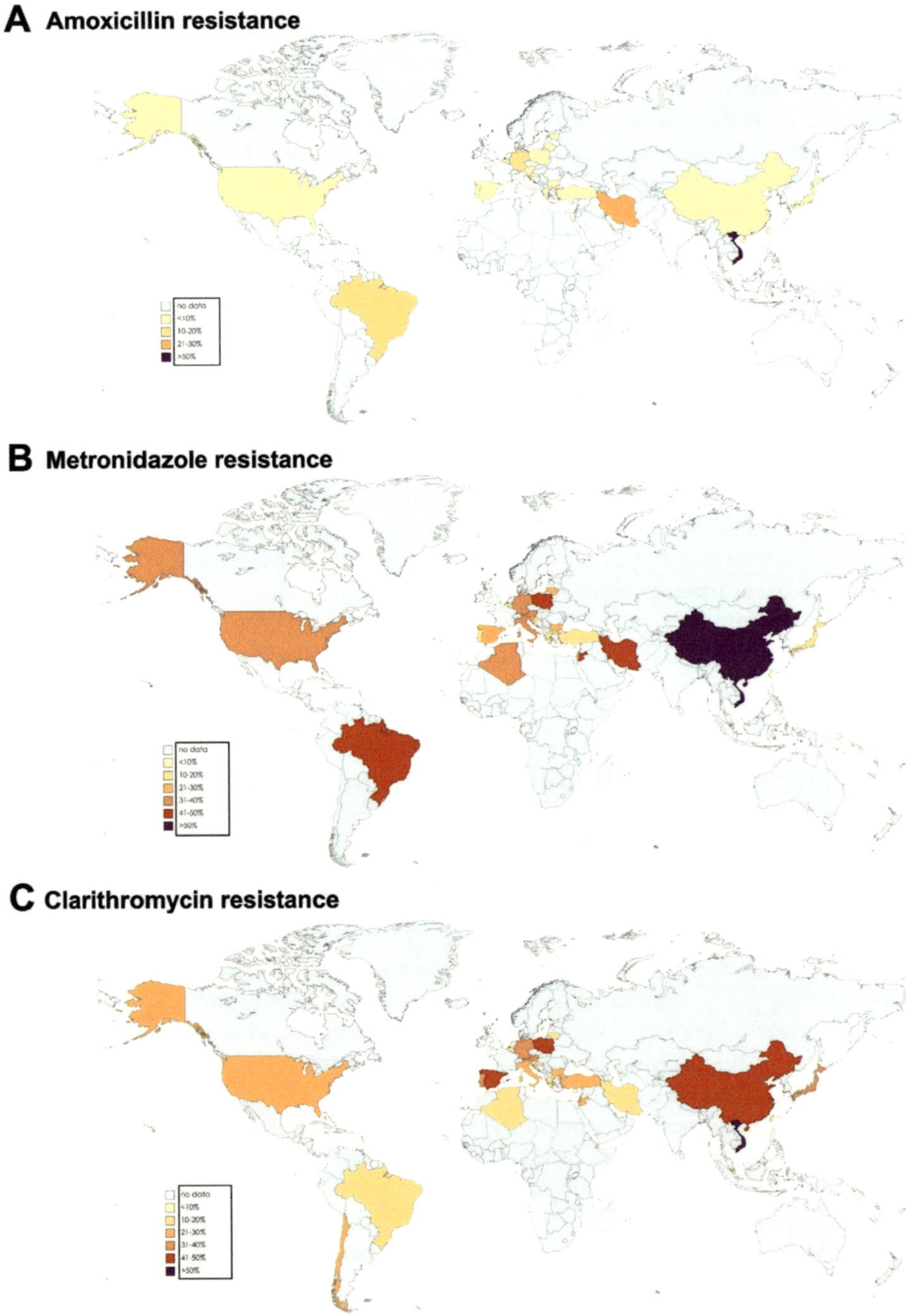

Figure 2.
Estimated pooled prevalence of antibiotic resistance for amoxicillin (A), metronidazole (B), and clarithromycin (C) of H. pylori among children from 28 countries in 5 WHO regions during (2000–2023).

clarithromycin and levofloxacin exhibit resistance rates of 46.1 and 44.0%, respectively, particularly among individuals under 40 years of age [38]. **Figure 2** illustrates the antibiotic resistance rates for metronidazole, amoxicillin, and clarithromycin within countries that have contributed their data on a global scale [39].

5. Clinical implications

The primary clinical consequence of antibiotic resistance in *H. pylori* is a significant reduction in the effectiveness of eradication treatment.

5.1 Treatment failures

The primary clinical implication of antibiotic resistance in *H. pylori* infection is the significant increase in treatment failures. Bacterial eradicate may result in persistent gastritis, complications of ulcer, and increased risk of gastric neoplasms. Health service providers need to consider local resistance standards when prescribing treatment regimes. For patients with known resistance, susceptibility tests can guide the choice of antibiotics, although availability is often limited [40].

Common causes:

1. Antibiotic resistance: *H. pylori* can develop resistance to often-used antibiotics, such as clarithromycin, metronidazole and levofloxacin. A study involving 1050 patients found a resistance rate of 24% for clarithromycin, 43.2% for metronidazole and 33.9% for levofloxacin [41].

2. Inadequate patient supporter: Failure to comply with prescribed treatment regimens significantly reduces the success of the extinction. Factors such as complex dosage plans and side effects can affect compliance [42].

5.2 Improving eradication treatment

It is recommended to apply treatment plans that are locally effective based on regional susceptibility patterns, since antibiotic resistance tendencies vary by geographic location [43]. To help with the selection of empirical eradication therapy, many countries, however, lack reliable information on the prevalence and characteristics of antibiotic resistance in local populations.

5.3 Alternative treatment approaches

Despite the resistance, alternative regimes were developed. Quadruple therapy containing bismuth subsalicylate, which combines bismuth subsalicylate with two antibiotics and a proton pump inhibitor, shows promise, particularly in regions with high resistance rates. Sequential therapy, in which different antibiotics are administered over time, is another strategy that can increase eradication rates [44].

5.4 Tailored therapy

Antibiotics are selected according to the antimicrobial susceptibility profile in tailored therapy, which is the best way to increase the effectiveness of *H. pylori* eradication treatment while reducing the number of unnecessary antibiotic prescriptions [45]. When the empirical regimen is quite successful in eliminating *H. pylori*, the advantage of tailored therapy is not obvious right away. Furthermore, this approach has been challenging due to the restricted availability of *H. pylori* cultures and antibiotic susceptibility testing [46].

5.5 Role of probiotics

Research indicates that integrating specific probiotic strains, such as Saccharomyces boulardii and certain Lactobacillus species, into standard antibiotic regimens can improve eradication rates while simultaneously reducing adverse effects associated with these treatments, thus highlighting their clinical significance in managing *H. pylori* infections [47, 48]. The mechanisms through which probiotics exert their beneficial effects in *H. pylori* therapy include immune modulation, enhancement of gut barrier function, and competitive exclusion of pathogenic bacteria.

These mechanisms contribute to an overall reduction in *H. pylori* colonization and improved gut health, which is essential for successful treatment outcomes [39, 49]. Clinical studies, including meta-analyses, have demonstrated that probiotic supplementation can significantly enhance eradication rates and mitigate side effects such as antibiotic-associated diarrhea, underscoring the value of probiotics as adjunctive therapies in *H. pylori* management [47, 48]. The role of probiotics in the eradication therapy of *H. pylori* infections is a growing area of interest that combines clinical relevance with ongoing research challenges.

6. Conclusion

Helicobacter pylori (*H. Pylori*) antibiotic resistance poses a significant challenge in global health, contributing to increase treatment failure rates and raising the risk of chronic gastric conditions such as peptic ulcers, mucosal-associated lymphoma (MALT) and gastric cancer. This chapter explores the primary resistance mechanisms, including punctual mutations in target genes, overexpression of efflux pumps and biofilm formation, each contributing to the reduction of antibiotic effectiveness. The growing prevalence of *H. pylori* resistant strains highlighted the urgent need for personalized treatment strategies, guided by antimicrobial susceptibility tests. In this context, resistance-guided therapy is increasingly favored in relation to empirical regimes. To address current therapeutic limitations, researchers are investigating new solutions, such as optimized combined therapies, probiotics as adjuvant treatments and the development of new antimicrobial agents more effectively. In addition, improving diagnostic accuracy through molecular methods can facilitate previous and more directed interventions. Future research should focus on overcoming diagnostic and therapeutic challenges, promoting antimicrobial administration and understanding regional resistance standards. A comprehensive and personalized approach is essential to achieve effective *H. pylori* eradication, reduce recurrence and minimize long-term load of global-scale infection. These efforts are vital to improving clinical results and containing the threat of antimicrobial resistance.

DOI: http://dx.doi.org/10.5772/intechopen.1010640

Author details

Kareem Ibraheem[1,2]*, Osama Hroub[1,2], Abdalrahman N. Herbawi[1] and Majed Dwaik[3]

1 Faculty of Medicine, Palestine Polytechnic University, Hebron, Palestine

2 Palestinian Clinical Research Center, Bethlehem, Palestine

3 College of Medicine and Health Sciences Palestine Polytechnic University, Hebron, Palestine

*Address all correspondence to: kareemjaberibraheem@gmail.com

References

[1] Borka Balas R, Meliț LE, Mărginean CO. Worldwide prevalence and risk factors of *Helicobacter pylori* infection in children. Children (Basel). 2022;**9**(9):1359. DOI: 10.3390/children9091359

[2] Bashir SK, Khan MB. Overview of *Helicobacter pylori* infection, prevalence, risk factors, and its prevention. Advanced Gut & Microbiome Research. 2023;**2023**:9747027. DOI: 10.1155/2023/9747027

[3] Fashner J, Gitu AC. Diagnosis and treatment of peptic ulcer disease and *H. Pylori* infection. American Family Physician. 2015;**91**(4):236-242

[4] Ali A, AlHussaini KI. *Helicobacter pylori*: A contemporary perspective on pathogenesis, diagnosis and treatment strategies. Microorganisms. 2024;**12**(1):222. DOI: 10.3390/microorganisms12010222

[5] Correa P, Piazuelo MB. *Helicobacter pylori* infection and gastric adenocarcinoma. US Gastroenterology and Hepatology Review. 2011;**7**(1):59-64

[6] Pereira MI, Medeiros JA. Role of *Helicobacter pylori* in gastric mucosa-associated lymphoid tissue lymphomas. World Journal of Gastroenterology. 2014;**20**(3):684-698. DOI: 10.3748/wjg.v20.i3.684

[7] Elbehiry A, Marzouk E, Aldubaib M, et al. *Helicobacter pylori* infection: Current status and future prospects on diagnostic, therapeutic and control challenges. Antibiotics (Basel). 2023;**12**(2):191. DOI: 10.3390/antibiotics12020191

[8] Malfertheiner P, Megraud F, O'Morain CA, et al. Management of *Helicobacter pylori* infection-the Maastricht V/Florence consensus report. Gut. 2017;**66**(1):6-30. DOI: 10.1136/gutjnl-2016-312288

[9] Malfertheiner P, Megraud F, O'Morain CA, et al. Management of *Helicobacter pylori* infection–the Maastricht IV/Florence consensus report. Gut. 2012;**61**(5):646-664. DOI: 10.1136/gutjnl-2012-302084

[10] Malfertheiner P, Megraud F, Rokkas T, et al. Management of *Helicobacter pylori* infection: The Maastricht VI/Florence consensus report. Gut. 2022;**71**(9):1724-1762. DOI: 10.1136/gutjnl-2022-327745

[11] Hu Y, Wan JH, Li XY, Zhu Y, Graham DY, Lu NH. Systematic review with meta-analysis: The global recurrence rate of *Helicobacter pylori*. Alimentary Pharmacology & Therapeutics. 2017;**46**(9):773-779. DOI: 10.1111/apt.14319

[12] Ford AC, Delaney BC, Forman D, Moayyedi P. Eradication therapy in *Helicobacter pylori* positive peptic ulcer disease: Systematic review and economic analysis. The American Journal of Gastroenterology. 2004;**99**(9):1833-1855. DOI: 10.1111/j.1572-0241.2004.40014.x

[13] Blaser MJ. Antibiotic use and its consequences for the normal microbiome. Science. 2016;**352**(6285):544-545. DOI: 10.1126/science.aad9358

[14] Sung JJY, Coker OO, Chu E, et al. Gastric microbes associated with gastric inflammation, atrophy and intestinal metaplasia 1 year after *Helicobacter pylori* eradication. Gut. 2020;**69**(9):1572-1580. DOI: 10.1136/gutjnl-2019-319826

[15] Wang Y, Du J, Zhang D, et al. Primary antibiotic resistance in *Helicobacter pylori* in China: A systematic review and meta-analysis. Journal of Global Antimicrobial Resistance. 2023;**34**:30-38. DOI: 10.1016/j.jgar.2023.05.014

[16] Savoldi A, Carrara E, Graham DY, Conti M, Tacconelli E. Prevalence of antibiotic resistance in *Helicobacter pylori*: A systematic review and meta-analysis in World Health Organization regions. Gastroenterology. 2018;**155**(5):1372-1382.e17. DOI: 10.1053/j.gastro.2018.07.007

[17] Ishibashi F, Suzuki S, Nagai M, Mochida K, Morishita T. Optimizing *Helicobacter pylori* treatment: An updated review of empirical and susceptibility test-based treatments. Gut Liver. 2023;**17**(5):684-697. DOI: 10.5009/gnl220429

[18] Thung I, Aramin H, Vavinskaya V, et al. Review article: The global emergence of *Helicobacter pylori* antibiotic resistance. Alimentary Pharmacology & Therapeutics. 2016;**43**(4):514-533. DOI: 10.1111/apt.13497

[19] Chey WD, Howden CW, Moss SF, et al. ACG clinical guideline: Treatment of *Helicobacter pylori* infection. The American Journal of Gastroenterology. 2024;**119**(9):1730-1753. DOI: 10.14309/ajg.0000000000002968

[20] World Health Organization. Global Antimicrobial Resistance and Use Surveillance System (GLASS) Report: 2021. Geneva: World Health Organization; 2021

[21] Hasanuzzaman M, Bang CS, Gong EJ. Antibiotic resistance of *Helicobacter pylori*: Mechanisms and clinical implications. Journal of Korean Medical Science. 2024;**39**(4):e44. DOI: 10.3346/jkms.2024.39.e44

[22] Ayaş M, Oktem-Okullu S, Özcan O, et al. Exploring the molecular mechanisms of macrolide resistance in laboratory mutant *Helicobacter pylori*. Antibiotics (Basel). 2024;**13**(5):396. DOI: 10.3390/antibiotics13050396

[23] Marques AT, Vítor JMB, Santos A, Oleastro M, Vale FF. Trends in *Helicobacter pylori* resistance to clarithromycin: From phenotypic to genomic approaches. Microbial Genomics. 2020;**6**(3):e000344. DOI: 10.1099/mgen.0.000344

[24] Bodunova N, Tsapkova L, Polyakova V, et al. Genetic markers of *Helicobacter pylori* resistance to clarithromycin and levofloxacin in Moscow, Russia. Current Issues in Molecular Biology. 2024;**46**(7):6665-6674. DOI: 10.3390/cimb46070397

[25] Zerbetto De Palma G, Mendiondo N, Wonaga A, et al. Occurrence of mutations in the antimicrobial target genes related to levofloxacin, clarithromycin, and amoxicillin resistance in *Helicobacter pylori* isolates from Buenos Aires city. Microbial Drug Resistance. 2017;**23**:351-358

[26] Zaki ME, Othman W, Ali MA, Shehta A. Fluoroquinolone-resistant *Helicobacter pylori* strains isolated from one Egyptian university hospital: Molecular aspects. Journal of Microbiology and Antimicrobial Agents (UK: Academy of Medical and Biological Sciences (AMBS)). 2016;**2**(1):26-31

[27] Hooi JKY, Lai WY, Ng WK, et al. Global prevalence of *Helicobacter pylori* infection: Systematic review and meta-analysis. Gastroenterology. 2017;**153**(2):420-429. DOI: 10.1053/j.gastro.2017.04.022

[28] Suerbaum S, Josenhans C. *Helicobacter pylori* evolution and

phenotypic diversification in a changing host. Nature Reviews. Microbiology. 2007;**5**(6):441-452. DOI: 10.1038/nrmicro1658

[29] Rocha GR, Lemos FFB, Silva LGO, et al. Overcoming antibiotic-resistant *Helicobacter pylori* infection: Current challenges and emerging approaches. World Journal of Gastroenterology. 2025;**31**(10):102289. DOI: 10.3748/wjg.v31.i10.102289

[30] Krzyżek P, Migdał P, Grande R, Gościniak G. Biofilm formation of *Helicobacter pylori* in both static and microfluidic conditions is associated with resistance to clarithromycin. Frontiers in Cellular and Infection Microbiology. 2022;**12**:868905. DOI: 10.3389/fcimb.2022.868905

[31] Vieira RR, Fontes LES, Pacheco RL, et al. Proton pump inhibitor- and clarithromycin-based triple therapies for *Helicobacter pylori* eradication. Cochrane Database of Systematic Reviews. 2020;**2020**(9):CD013734. DOI: 10.1002/14651858.CD013734

[32] Nista EC, Pellegrino A, Giuli L, et al. Clinical implications of *Helicobacter pylori* antibiotic resistance in Italy: A review of the literature. Antibiotics (Basel). 2022;**11**(10):1452. DOI: 10.3390/antibiotics11101452

[33] Boyanova L, Hadzhiyski P, Gergova R, Markovska R. Evolution of *Helicobacter pylori* resistance to antibiotics: A topic of increasing concern. Antibiotics (Basel). 2023;**12**(2):332. DOI: 10.3390/antibiotics12020332

[34] Lin Y, Shao Y, Yan J, Ye G. Antibiotic resistance in *Helicobacter pylori*: From potential biomolecular mechanisms to clinical practice. Journal of Clinical Laboratory Analysis. 2023;**37**(7):e24885. DOI: 10.1002/jcla.24885

[35] Gisbert JP. Rifabutin for the treatment of *Helicobacter pylori* infection: A review. Pathogens. 2020;**10**(1):15. DOI: 10.3390/pathogens10010015

[36] Mégraud F. *H. pylori* antibiotic resistance: Prevalence, importance, and advances in testing. Gut. 2004;**53**(9):1374-1384. DOI: 10.1136/gut.2003.022111

[37] Nestegard O, Moayeri B, Halvorsen FA, et al. *Helicobacter pylori* resistance to antibiotics before and after treatment: Incidence of eradication failure. PLoS One. 2022;**17**(4):e0265322. DOI: 10.1371/journal.pone.0265322

[38] Deng R, Liu L, Xie W, et al. Prevalence of *Helicobacter pylori* antibiotic resistance in patients enrolled in Guangzhou, China. Infection and Drug Resistance. 2023;**16**:5033-5038. DOI: 10.2147/IDR.S418482

[39] Salahi-Niri A, Nabavi-Rad A, Monaghan TM, et al. Global prevalence of *Helicobacter pylori* antibiotic resistance among children in the World Health Organization regions between 2000 and 2023: A systematic review and meta-analysis. BMC Medicine. 2024;**22**:598. DOI: 10.1186/s12916-024-03816-y

[40] Zhang M. High antibiotic resistance rate: A difficult issue for *Helicobacter pylori* eradication treatment. World Journal of Gastroenterology. 2015;**21**(48):13432-13437. DOI: 10.3748/wjg.v21.i48.13432

[41] Aumpan N, Issariyakulkarn N, Mahachai V, et al. Management of *Helicobacter pylori* treatment failures: A large population-based study (HP treatment failures trial). PLoS One. 2023;**18**(11):e0294403. DOI: 10.1371/journal.pone.0294403

[42] O'Connor JP, Taneike I, O'Morain C. Improving compliance with *Helicobacter*

pylori eradication therapy: When and how? Therapeutic Advances in Gastroenterology. 2009;**2**(5):273-279. DOI: 10.1177/1756283X09337342

[43] Shiotani A, Roy P, Lu H, Graham DY. *Helicobacter pylori* diagnosis and therapy in the era of antimicrobial stewardship. Therapeutic Advances in Gastroenterology. 2021;**14**:17562848211064080. DOI: 10.1177/17562848211064080

[44] Salam MA, Al-Amin MY, Salam MT, et al. Antimicrobial resistance: A growing serious threat for global public health. Healthcare (Basel). 2023;**11**(13):1946. DOI: 10.3390/healthcare11131946

[45] Bae JH, Jo HH, Kwon JG, Kim EY. Efficacy of 7-day tailored therapy for *Helicobacter pylori* eradication based on clarithromycin resistance. The Korean Journal of Gastroenterology. 2023;**82**(1):10-17. DOI: 10.4166/kjg.2023.039

[46] Nyssen OP, Espada M, Gisbert JP. Empirical vs. susceptibility-guided treatment of *Helicobacter pylori* infection: A systematic review and meta-analysis. Frontiers in Microbiology. 2022;**13**:913436. DOI: 10.3389/fmicb.2022.913436

[47] Wang Y, Wang X, Cao XY, et al. Comparative effectiveness of different probiotics supplements for triple *Helicobacter pylori* eradication: A network meta-analysis. Frontiers in Cellular and Infection Microbiology. 2023;**13**:1120789. DOI: 10.3389/fcimb.2023.1120789

[48] Tanashat M, Abuelazm M, Abouzid M, et al. Efficacy of probiotics regimens for *Helicobacter pylori* eradication: A systematic review, pairwise, and network meta-analysis of randomized controlled trials. Clinical Nutrition ESPEN. 2025;**65**:424-444. DOI: 10.1016/j.clnesp.2024.11.016

[49] Keikha M, Karbalaei M. Probiotics as the live microscopic fighters against *Helicobacter pylori* gastric infections. BMC Gastroenterology. 2021;**21**(1):388. DOI: 10.1186/s12876-021-01977-1

Chapter 5

H. pylori and Herpesviruses: "Commonwealth" or "Every Man for Himself"

Gulustan H. Babayeva, Umud R. Mahmudov, Jamal S. Musayev, Ferid V. Guliyev, Emin Kh. Verdiyev, Rashad A. Hasanov, Gunay V. Asadova, Rafail H. Hasanov, Aychin I. Hasanova and Nargiz E. Afandiyeva

Abstract

Infections caused by *Helicobacter pylori* and human herpesviruses are important links in the pathogenesis of inflammatory and neoplastic diseases of the upper gastrointestinal tract. Infection with this microorganism is associated with the development of chronic gastritis, gastric and duodenal ulcer, atrophic and metaplastic mucosal changes, and in some cases, gastric adenocarcinoma and MALT lymphoma. In addition, herpesviruses, especially the Epstein-Barr virus and cytomegalovirus, are highly prevalent among the adult population and can persist in the body throughout life. They have a tropism for epithelial and immune cells and, like *H. pylori*, can cause chronic inflammation, disrupt the regulation of apoptosis and the cell cycle, activate oncogenic signaling pathways, and induce epigenetic changes in the gastric mucosa. Modern studies increasingly point to the possibility of coinfection with *H. pylori* and herpesviruses, which can enhance the inflammatory response, aggravate damage to the mucosa, and increase the risk of transformation of a benign process into a malignant one. In particular, signs of the simultaneous presence of both bacterial and viral pathogens are increasingly found in foci of chronic gastritis, peptic ulcer disease, and precancerous changes in the gastro-duodenal mucosa. Thus, the study of the interaction of *H. pylori* and herpesviruses in the gastro-duodenal mucosa is an important direction in understanding the pathogenesis of gastrointestinal diseases. This allows not only to clarify the mechanisms of inflammation and carcinogenesis but also to reconsider approaches to diagnostics, treatment, and prevention of these conditions.

Keywords: *Helicobacter pylori*, human herpesviruses, Epstein-Barr (EBV HHV-4), cytomegalovirus (CMV HHV-5), inflammation, gastric cancer

1. Introduction

Helicobacter pylori (*H. pylori*) is one of the most significant bacterial pathogens of humans, possessing a unique ability for long-term colonization of the gastric mucosa. This gram-negative spiral-shaped bacterium has adapted to the aggressive acidic environment of the stomach due to the production of urease, changes in the pH of the microenvironment, and the ability to form biofilms. According to global epidemiological studies, *H. pylori* infects more than 50% of the world's population, while the prevalence rate varies from 20 to 30% in economically developed countries to 70–90% in developing regions. Chronic *H. pylori* infection is the main etiologic factor in the development of chronic gastritis, gastric ulcer, and duodenal ulcer, as well as precancerous conditions—atrophic gastritis and intestinal metaplasia—preceding gastric adenocarcinoma. The International Agency for Research on Cancer (IARC) has classified *H. pylori* as a Group 1 carcinogen. Growing evidence also points to a role for *H. pylori* in extragastric pathologies, including idiopathic thrombocytopenic purpura, iron deficiency anemia, atherosclerosis, and neurodegenerative diseases.

Human herpesviruses (family Herpesviridae) are a group of deoxyribonucleic acid (DNA) viruses that include eight pathogens that infect humans: herpes simplex viruses types 1 and 2 (HSV-1/HSV-2), varicella-zoster virus (VZV), cytomegalovirus (CMV), and Epstein-Barr virus (EBV), as well as HHV-6, HHV-7, and HHV-8 (associated with Kaposi's sarcoma). All members of the family have a key feature—the ability to have latent persistence in the body and reactivation when the host's immune status changes. In recent years, more and more studies have shown that herpesviruses can be detected in the gastric mucosa, especially in patients with chronic gastritis, peptic ulcer disease, and immunodeficiency states.

The interaction of *H. pylori* and herpes viruses is considered a new important aspect of the pathogenesis of diseases of the upper gastrointestinal tract. The joint persistence of these pathogens can enhance chronic inflammation due to:

- modulation of the innate and adaptive immune response, including activation of the Th1/Th17 pathways and depletion of regulatory mechanisms;
- enhancement of the cytokine cascade (increased production of IL-1β, IL-6, and TNF-α), which leads to damage to the epithelium;
- changes in the barrier function of the mucosa, increased permeability, and imbalance of the microbiota;
- reactivation of herpes viruses against the background of inflammation, which can maintain chronic tissue damage and precancerous changes.

Current data indicate that coinfection with *H. pylori* and herpesviruses (especially EBV and CMV) is associated with a more severe course of gastritis, resistance to eradication therapy, and, probably, an increased risk of neoplastic processes. A number of studies have shown that EBV can infect gastric epithelial cells, forming a special variant of EBV-positive adenocarcinoma, while CMV is able to modulate the immune response and potentiate chronic inflammation. Thus, the study of the combined effect of *H. pylori* and herpesviruses opens up new prospects for understanding the pathogenesis of chronic inflammatory and neoplastic processes in the stomach and duodenum. This direction is important for the development of new diagnostic algorithms, personalized treatment strategies (including combined eradication regimens), and primary prevention measures in risk groups.

Helicobacter pylori (*H. pylori*) and viruses of the Herpesviridae family are two different pathogens that can cause disease in humans, and they differ significantly in their nature and mechanisms of action, but certain relationships and interactions may exist between them.

Helicobacter pylori is a gram-negative bacterium that colonizes the mucous membrane of the stomach and duodenum. It is one of the main causes of gastric and duodenal ulcers, as well as chronic gastritis. The presence of *H. pylori* is associated with an increased risk of developing stomach cancer, since long-term inflammation of the mucous membrane can lead to pathological changes in the tissues. The infection is usually transmitted by the fecal-oral route and can persist in the body for years, causing chronic inflammation.

The Herpesviridae family includes many viruses that can infect humans, the most well-known of which are herpes simplex viruses (HSV-1 and HSV-2), herpes type 3 (varicella-zoster virus (VZV)), herpes type 4 (Epstein-Barr virus), herpes type 5 (cytomegalovirus), and herpes types 6, 7, and 8.

Thus, *Helicobacter pylori* and Herpesviridae viruses differ in their biological nature—one is a bacterium, the others are viruses—as well as in their transmission routes and clinical manifestations. However, their joint presence in the body can affect the course of diseases, which requires further research to understand the possible interactions between these pathogens [1, 2].

In addition, herpes viruses can cause other less common diseases such as keratitis and encephalitis, especially in people with weakened immune systems [3].

2. Herpes simplex virus 1 and 2

HSV-1 primarily causes oral herpes, which manifests as painful blisters and ulcers on the lips and around the mouth. HSV-2, in turn, is more often associated with genital herpes. Herpes simplex virus 1 is a double-stranded DNA virus that is transmitted primarily through saliva, as well as by direct contact with infected mucous membranes or skin. After the primary infection, the virus remains latent in the body, periodically causing relapses of the disease. HSV-1 is constantly present in the body in a dormant state in ganglion cells and can periodically reactivate [4]. Herpes virus infections are widespread among humans. Serological studies show that most adults (up to 95%) are infected [5, 6]. Moreover, this infection can be asymptomatic, which contributes to the high prevalence of HSV-1 infection worldwide [7].

3. Varicella-zoster virus (VZV)

Varicella-zoster virus (also known as human herpesvirus type 3) is the cause of both chickenpox and shingles. Chickenpox usually occurs during a primary infection, most often in childhood, after which the virus remains in the body in an inactive (latent) form in nerve cells. Subsequent reactivation of the virus, usually due to a weakened immune system, can result in shingles. It is characterized by a one-sided rash and painful lesions, often with pain along the nerves. Factors that contribute to the reactivation of the virus include weakened immunity, stress, chronic diseases, and old age (especially over 50 years).

4. Human herpesvirus type 4: Epstein-Barr virus (EBV)

Known as the cause of infectious mononucleosis and associated with some cancers [8].

Epstein-Barr virus (EBV) causes a widespread infection worldwide, affecting more than 90% of the adult population [9]. This is due to its ability to establish lifelong latency with episodes of reactivation in the absence of major clinical symptoms in most cases. EBV is a member of the Herpesviridae, sharing the main characteristics of herpes infections—persistence, latency, and reactivation. It has been associated with various malignancies, and some evidence suggests that EBV reactivations may alter the natural history of other coinfections [10]. Chronic herpes infections, including EBV, may accelerate immune aging, directly impacting lifespan [11].

What is more interesting is the clinical manifestations of concomitant and sequential infections and reactivations of EBV and other pathogens. It is believed that concomitant infection is usually possible due to similar pathways and is associated with more severe disease. However, the subsequent infectious agent may find the host in an immunocompetent state. EBV usually attacks the entire immune system and usually results in a stable immune response.

5. Human herpesvirus type 5 (HHV-5)-cytomegalovirus (CMV)

Cytomegalovirus (CMV) is a common virus from the herpesvirus family (human herpesvirus type 5), which is often asymptomatic in people with normal immunity but can cause serious diseases in people with weakened immune systems, newborns, and pregnant women. CMV is transmitted through biological fluids: blood, saliva, milk, urine, seminal fluid, and cervical secretions. CMV remains in the body for life. In healthy people, the infection is often asymptomatic or causes mild flu-like symptoms.

Symptoms of primary infection (in adults): temperature up to 38°C, general and muscle weakness, enlarged cervical lymph nodes, headache, discomfort in the salivary glands, sore throat, and runny nose.

It is dangerous for vulnerable groups: people with weakened immune systems (HIV-infected and transplant recipients) can suffer severe organ damage (pneumonia, hepatitis, chorioretinitis, and damage to the esophagus and intestines).

In pregnant women, it can lead to congenital malformations in the fetus, and in newborns, it is the most common cause of congenital malformations in industrialized countries.

It is classified by the timing and mechanisms of infection (congenital, acquired), the degree of virus activity (latent, active), and the type of infection (primary, reactivation, reinfection).

6. Herpes simplex virus type 6 (HHV-6)

A DNA virus of the Herpesviridae family that primarily affects immune cells, bone marrow, liver, and the nervous system is often asymptomatic but can cause a variety of manifestations, including roseola infantum (sudden exanthema), flu-like symptoms, mononucleosis-like syndrome, and complications with reduced immunity.

There are two subtypes—HHV-6A and HHV-6B. HHV-6 is widespread in the human population, and the first infection usually occurs in early childhood.

The infection is transmitted by airborne droplets, contact-household, and transplacental routes, with saliva and sputum being the main transmission factors.

After the initial infection, the virus persists in the body for life in a latent form, mainly by integrating the genome into the chromosomes of the host cells, which makes diagnosis difficult.

Clinical manifestations: The course is mostly asymptomatic, and most people are infected without any symptoms.

Roseola infantum (sudden exanthema, sixth disease): The most common symptom in children, characterized by high fever, which after 3–4 days is replaced by a rash all over the body, usually without itching.

Some people may develop flu-like symptoms: fever, headache, fatigue, and muscle and joint pain.

May manifest as a mononucleosis-like syndrome, accompanied by fatigue, enlarged lymph nodes, liver and spleen, and sore throat. People with weakened immune systems, such as those with HIV infection or organ transplants, may develop more severe conditions, including encephalitis, myocarditis, pneumonia, bone marrow suppression, and immunodeficiencies.

The virus is neurotropic, infecting immune cells as well as the bone marrow, liver, skin, and nervous system.

7. Relationships between herpesviruses and *Helicobacter pylori*

It has previously been suggested that EBV infection may play a protective role for other types of infections [12]. The same divergence of ideas and controversies can be observed in the literature on the role of *Helicobacter pylori*. There are quite a few studies showing a protective role of non-eradicated *H. pylori* infection in various autoimmune diseases [13]. Could the same be true for HSV and perhaps other herpesviruses? Below is a study based mainly on two hypotheses about the potential protective role of ongoing *H. pylori* infection against the manifestation of herpes infection. The authors tested sera from 190 dental patients (mean age 52 years) who underwent an oral examination. Clinical findings included general oral pathology and superficial oral lesions. Exclusion criteria were malignant neoplasms of the maxillofacial region, as well as the presence of other malignant neoplasms.

8. EBV and *H. pylori*

The authors performed serological tests to determine EBV and *H. pylori* infection; more than 90% of the participants had evidence of previous infection (27% had a fairly high titer (>750 U/ml) of EBV VCA IgG). Serological testing for *H. pylori* was performed in 64 participants, with a positive result in 55% of cases (35/64). The results of laboratory testing are presented below in **Figure 1** [8].

The authors suggested that in people with a strong humoral immune response to EBV, *H. pylori* infection occurs less frequently—25% versus 65% ($p < 0.01$).

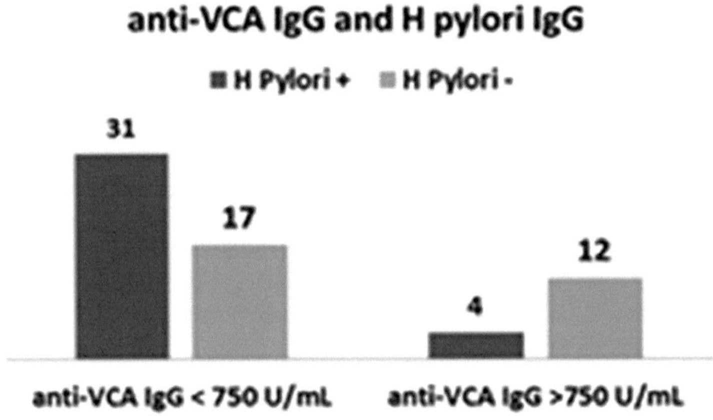

Figure 1.
Anti-VCA IgG and H. pylori *(adapted from Krasteva and Petrova [8]).*

9. HSV1/2 and *H. pylori*

The authors further identified serological evidence of acute HSV infection in 18% of patients (126 participants). *H. pylori* was positive in 56% of the 88 tested, regardless of age and gender. The results of diagnostics for *H. pylori* showed that the overall serological prevalence of HSV was 13% and that of *H. pylori* was 57%. Patients without signs of HSV2 were *H. pylori*-positive in 63% of cases, while none of the HSV2-positive patients were *H. pylori*-positive (p = 0.0046, Fisher). The authors concluded that acute HSV2 infection is more often detected in individuals with a negative result for *H. pylori* (**Figure 2**) [8].

When analyzing the data, it was noted that patients with acute herpes simplex virus type 1 (HSV-1) infection were significantly less likely to have *Helicobacter pylori* infection compared to the group without HSV-1 (1 of 8 versus 33 of 52, p = 0.0164 by Fisher's test) (see **Figure 3**) [8].

This result raises an interesting question about whether *H. pylori* may have a protective effect against other infections. Several studies have previously examined

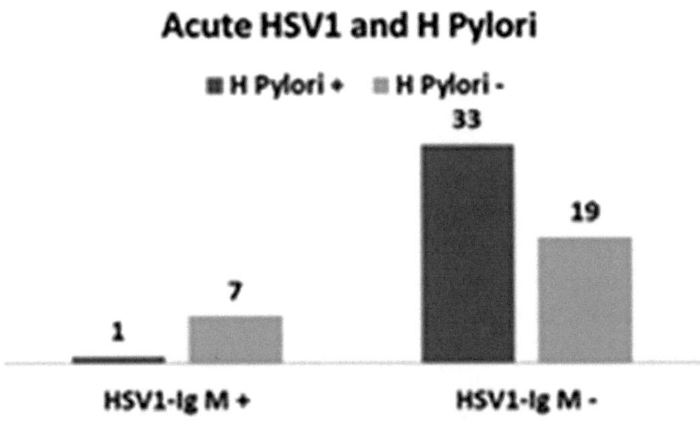

Figure 2.
Acute HSV2 and H. pylori *(adapted from Krasteva and Petrova [8]).*

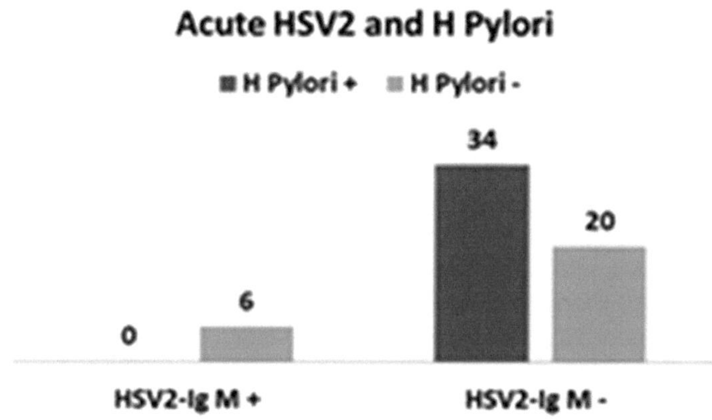

Figure 3.
Acute HSV1 and H. pylori *(adapted from Krasteva and Petrova [8]).*

the interactions between viruses and bacteria in the gastric mucosa. For example, in patients with peptic ulcer disease, the presence of HSV-1 was associated with a lower likelihood of *H. pylori* infection. In addition, a study of the adult population in Greece found an inverse association between HSV-1 and *H. pylori* infections, indicating a possible mutual influence of these microorganisms and their role in shaping the microbial ecology of the mucosa [14]. In contrast to the above findings, a study among adolescents in the United States found the opposite trend: seropositivity for herpes simplex virus type 1 (HSV-1) was associated with a higher rate of seropositivity for *Helicobacter pylori*. The authors of this study did not find any obvious biological mechanisms that could explain this association between the two infections. Therefore, it was suggested that this coincidence may be due to common routes of transmission of these pathogens. For example, both microorganisms can be transmitted through contact with contaminated secretions or the fecal-oral route, which is especially common in settings with poor hygiene. In addition, socioeconomic and demographic factors, such as poor sanitation or population density, may favor the co-occurrence of both infections in certain populations. Thus, these findings highlight the complexity of interactions between viruses and bacteria and the need to consider the context of epidemiological factors when interpreting coinfection data [15]. The above results demonstrated opposite relationships between infections, which may reflect the influence of local immune interactions or more complex mechanisms of the host immune response. Such differences in correlations suggest that the interaction between *Helicobacter pylori* and herpes simplex virus type 1 (HSV-1) is not straightforward and may depend on multiple factors, including features of immune regulation at the mucosal membranes, the state of the microbiota, and individual characteristics of the organism. These data highlight the importance of further research to elucidate the mechanisms underlying such relationships, which may have implications for understanding the pathogenesis and developing new approaches to the prevention and treatment of infectious diseases.

Over the past decade, coinfection with *Helicobacter pylori* and Epstein-Barr virus (EBV) has attracted increasing interest from researchers, especially in the context of its possible role in the pathogenesis of malignant neoplasms of the stomach. The involvement of EBV in the development of gastric carcinoma is actively discussed in the scientific literature, with *H. pylori* continuing to be considered a key etiological factor. However, increasing evidence suggests that EBV may also play a significant role in the formation of precancerous changes in the gastric mucosa. Although the effect of EBV on chronic gastric inflammation has been studied much less, some studies raise the hypothesis that the virus can initiate or enhance the inflammatory process, especially in the presence of coinfection with *H. pylori*. A number of studies suggest that EBV can act synergistically with *H. pylori*, increasing damage to the gastric epithelium, contributing to the disruption of tissue regeneration, and forming a stable inflammatory background. This chronic inflammatory process, maintained by both pathogens, may serve as a basis for further molecular changes predisposing to the development of malignant transformation of gastric epithelial cells. Thus, coinfection is considered a potentially important factor in the early stages of carcinogenesis [16]. Both pathogens, *Helicobacter pylori* and Epstein-Barr virus (EBV), are capable of modulating similar intracellular signaling pathways, resulting in activation of cell proliferation processes, increased survival of infected cells, and decreased efficiency of the body's immune response. These mechanisms contribute to the creation of a microenvironment favorable for chronic inflammation and subsequent oncogenesis. Interesting data were presented in a recent study by Saju P et al., which showed that cellular phosphatase SHP1 expressed in gastric epithelium performs a protective function, preventing the pathological action of CagA, one of the key virulence factors of *H. pylori*. However, the Epstein-Barr virus is capable of disrupting this protective function. In particular, when infecting gastric epithelial cells, EBV induces hypermethylation of the SHP1 gene promoter, which leads to epigenetic suppression of its expression. This decrease in SHP1 levels, in turn, enhances the phosphorylation-mediated action of CagA and may contribute to a more aggressive course of infection and increased proliferative and transformative processes in cells. These data highlight the importance of epigenetic mechanisms in the pathogenesis of coinfection and the possible synergy between *H. pylori* and EBV in gastric carcinogenesis [17]. While *H. pylori* promotes carcinogenesis primarily through epigenetic silencing of tumor suppressor genes, disrupting key regulatory mechanisms of cellular signaling pathways, EBV-associated tumors are characterized by an extensive and specific DNA hypermethylation profile. Such hypermethylation, observed in EBV-positive gastric carcinomas, affects the promoter regions of multiple genes, including those responsible for cell cycle control, apoptosis, and immune surveillance, which may contribute to the persistent suppression of antitumor mechanisms at the molecular level [18]. In addition to its role in gastric carcinogenesis, the interaction between *Helicobacter pylori* and the Epstein-Barr virus (EBV) is also becoming an object of active study in the context of peptic ulcer disease. Results of a recent serological study conducted in Mexico revealed a significant association between peptic ulcer disease and elevated levels of IgG antibodies to EBV. Moreover, the presence of IgA antibodies to EBV was positively associated with gastric ulcer, which may indicate localized activation of the virus in the gastric mucosa. Additional data show that EBV reactivation in epithelial cells of the stomach and duodenum can significantly increase the risk of developing ulcers—by some estimates, this risk increases tenfold. These results emphasize the importance of viral-bacterial interactions in the pathogenesis of not only malignant but also benign diseases of the gastrointestinal tract [19]. Interestingly, the results of the abovementioned study indicate a possible inverse relationship between *H. pylori* infection and a high serological response to EBV. In particular, it was found that elevated titers of antibodies to the Epstein-Barr virus are associated with a higher probability of a negative result for *H. pylori*. One of the possible mechanisms for this phenomenon is the activation of local immune responses that can limit the colonization of the gastric mucosa by *H. pylori*, as demonstrated in the study by Cárdenas-Mondragón et al. The findings highlight the need to reconsider the traditional clinical approach to the diagnosis and treatment of *H. pylori*. Given its long-term coexistence with the human population for thousands of years, *H. pylori* should be considered not only as a pathogen but also as a component of a complex gastric ecosystem interacting with other microorganisms and viruses. This requires a more comprehensive and individualized approach to its assessment in clinical practice [20]. Current approaches to the diagnosis and treatment of *Helicobacter pylori* may need to be revised, taking into account the possible coexistence of other infectious agents, including viruses. Further studies are needed to study the interactions between *H. pylori* and concomitant infections, since such interactions can significantly affect both the course of diseases and the effectiveness of therapeutic interventions. The authors emphasize that the interpretation of the results should take into account certain limitations of the study: a relatively small sample of patients, the lack of uniform criteria for serological assessment of Epstein-Barr virus reactivation, as well as the potential impact of cross-immune reactions on serological parameters. Nevertheless, the study of interpathogenic interactions is of great interest not only for fundamental science but also for clinical practice. Particular attention should be paid to the characteristics of coinfections with *H. pylori* and herpes viruses, not only in the context of oncogenesis but also in the context of more common, benign gastrointestinal diseases such as gastritis and peptic ulcer disease. The question remains whether *H. pylori* can exert a protective effect in the context of herpes virus infection or, conversely, whether an active immune response to the virus prevents colonization of the stomach by *H. pylori*. Larger, multicenter studies involving both immunological and microbiological approaches are needed to answer these questions.

Epstein-Barr virus (EBV) is a widespread member of the human herpesvirus family. Primary EBV infection may present as infectious mononucleosis and subsequently be associated with the development of malignant and autoimmune diseases such as Burkitt's lymphoma, nasopharyngeal carcinoma, systemic autoimmune disorders, and gastric cancer (GC). The persistent (latent) form of infection can cause the transformation of both lymphoid and epithelial cells, promoting the development of neoplasms due to disruption of cell cycle regulation, evasion of immune surveillance, and epigenetic changes. *Helicobacter pylori*, in turn, is a bacterium that can colonize the human gastric mucosa, causing chronic gastritis. This inflammatory condition often persists for many years and is considered a key factor contributing to the development of precancerous changes such as atrophy, intestinal metaplasia, and dysplasia. It is believed that long-term chronic inflammation induced by *H. pylori* plays an important role in the formation of genomic instability, which creates conditions for the accumulation of mutations and, ultimately, malignant transformation of cells. It is estimated that about 45% of the world's population is potentially infected with both *Helicobacter pylori* and Epstein-Barr virus (EBV), which emphasizes the relevance of studying their combined impact on human health. Approximately 180 people out of every 100,000 in the population develop gastric cancer (GC), which is often accompanied by various precancerous conditions and morphological abnormalities of the mucous membrane. These epidemiological indicators make gastric cancer the third leading cause of cancer-related deaths globally.

Despite the large number of studies investigating *H. pylori* and EBV separately, data on coinfection with these two pathogens remain extremely limited. However, the results of recently published studies suggest that coinfection with *H. pylori* and EBV may significantly increase the risk of gastric cancer development and be associated with an earlier age of disease manifestation compared to mono infection. This indicates a possible synergistic effect of coinfection on carcinogenesis and progression of gastric pathology [21].

10. Gastric cancer drivers: EBV and *Helicobacter pylori* coinfection

The interaction between Epstein-Barr virus (EBV) and *Helicobacter pylori* in the gastric mucosa may play a key role in the pathogenesis of gastric cancer (GC), potentially synergizing with the molecular mechanisms of carcinogenesis. Coinfection with these two pathogens can enhance the inflammatory response, disrupt cell cycle regulation, and promote epigenetic changes, including hypermethylation of tumor suppressor gene promoters. Analysis of tumor samples from gastric adenocarcinomas associated with EBV and *H. pylori* coinfection revealed an extensive hypermethylation profile of several key genes. The most frequently altered genes include COX-2 (cyclooxygenase-2), DAPK (cell death-associated kinase), CDH1 (encodes the protein E-cadherin, important for cell adhesion), CDKN2A (cyclin-dependent kinase inhibitor, regulating the cell cycle), and hMLH1 (involved in DNA repair). These genes are often involved in various types of malignancies, including gastric cancer, and their epigenetic inactivation is considered an important step in tumor initiation and progression. The accumulation of such molecular alterations in the presence of coinfection indicates a possible enhanced carcinogenic potential of the interaction of EBV and *H. pylori*, which requires further study and may have diagnostic and prognostic value [22]. In addition, patients with a positive *Helicobacter pylori* result have a significantly higher viral load of Epstein-Barr virus (EBV) DNA in gastric tissue. This fact may indicate a possible role of *H. pylori* in the activation of the EBV lytic cycle. It is assumed that bacterial infection promotes the transition of EBV from a latent state to a lytic phase, accompanied by active viral replication and increased pathogenetic effects on gastric epithelial cells. Such reactivation can increase the inflammatory process and tissue damage, contributing to carcinogenesis [23]. In addition, patients with gastric cancer infected with *Helicobacter pylori* had significantly higher levels of Epstein-Barr virus (EBV) DNA compared to patients not infected with *H. pylori*. These data suggest that the presence of *H. pylori* may promote enhanced EBV replication or reactivation in gastric tissue, thereby enhancing the oncogenic effect of the virus in the development of gastric cancer [24]. The results of a recent study on the coinfection of *Helicobacter pylori* and Epstein-Barr virus (EBV) indicate that the simultaneous presence of these pathogens in the gastric mucosa can cause pronounced inflammatory changes. The researchers suggest that such coinfection not only enhances the local immune response but also causes an imbalance of proinflammatory and anti-inflammatory cytokines, creating a stable microenvironment of chronic inflammation. Under conditions of constant immune stimulation, the epithelial barrier is damaged, signaling pathways involved in cell proliferation and survival are activated, and epigenetic changes are enhanced. All these processes create the prerequisites for the development of malignant transformation, especially toward intestinal-type adenocarcinoma. This histological subtype of gastric cancer often develops against the background of chronic gastritis, intestinal metaplasia, and dysplasia—conditions closely associated with long-term inflammation. Thus, coinfection with EBV and *H. pylori* may act as an important synergistic factor that significantly increases the risk of developing intestinal-type gastric cancer compared to isolated infection with each pathogen [20]. At least two pathogenetic mechanisms are proposed to explain the enhanced carcinogenic effect of *Helicobacter pylori* and Epstein-Barr virus (EBV) coinfection. The first mechanism is associated with the additional inflammatory load resulting from the simultaneous presence of both pathogens. Coinfection enhances innate and adaptive immune responses, leading to chronic inflammation and progressive damage to the gastric mucosa. Under conditions of constant activation of the immune system, the production of proinflammatory cytokines (such as IL-1β, IL-6, and TNF-α) and reactive oxygen species increases, which contributes to DNA damage, disruption of intercellular contacts, and activation of signaling pathways involved in cellular proliferation and survival. This inflammatory microenvironment, supported by *H. pylori* and EBV coinfection, not only enhances epithelial destruction but also creates conditions conducive to the accumulation of genetic and epigenetic changes, which increase the risk of malignant transformation [25, 26]. In this variant, the leading aspects were significant increases in the levels of IL-1β [27], TNF-α [28], and IL-8 [29]. One study conducted among pediatric patients showed that *Helicobacter pylori* itself is not associated with a pronounced inflammatory response. In contrast, the presence of Epstein-Barr virus (EBV) turned out to be a key factor associated with the development of severe inflammation of the gastric mucosa. These data suggest that in the pediatric population, EBV may play a leading role in the formation of a pronounced immune response and damage to the gastric epithelium, while *H. pylori* in monoinfection conditions does not cause such pronounced changes [20]. The second mechanism suggests that the interaction of EBV and *Helicobacter pylori* gene products, leading to activation of common signaling pathways, plays a decisive role in the pathogenesis of coinfection. In particular, it has been shown that reactivation of latent Epstein-Barr virus can occur through activation of the phospholipase C gamma (PLCγ) signaling pathway, which triggers expression of viral genes and transition of the virus to the lytic phase. At the same time, the virulence factor of *H. pylori*, the CagA protein, has the ability to actively activate the PLCγ pathway in infected gastric epithelial cells. Thus, CagA-*H. pylori*-mediated stimulation of PLCγ can promote EBV reactivation in gastric tissue. This interaction enhances viral replication, increases the production of viral proteins, and promotes further disruption of cellular regulation. Given that EBV reactivation is associated with increased inflammation, cytopathic effects, and potential for epithelial cell transformation, synergy between CagA and EBV within the PLCγ-signaling pathway may be considered an important molecular mechanism contributing to the progression of gastric pathology and carcinogenesis [30, 31]. Data obtained in experimental models confirm the oncogenic potential of CagA, one of the key virulence factors of *Helicobacter pylori*. In particular, studies on transgenic mice have shown that ectopic expression of the CagA gene leads to the development of proliferative disorders and tumor-like changes in various tissues, which confirms its nature as a bacterial oncoprotein. Such mice exhibit hyperplasia, dysplasia, and malignant transformation of the epithelium, especially in the gastrointestinal tract, which indicates the direct participation of CagA in the initiation of carcinogenesis [32–35].

CagA, the major oncoprotein of *Helicobacter pylori*, and the latent membrane proteins LMP1 and LMP2 of the Epstein-Barr virus (EBV) play a key role in activating cellular signaling pathways that promote cell survival and proliferation. In particular, all three proteins are capable of activating NF-κB and MAPK (mitogen-activated protein kinase) cascades, signaling pathways widely known for their role in the regulation of inflammation, cell proliferation, suppression of apoptosis, and tumor development. Activation of NF-κB leads to the transcription of genes encoding anti-inflammatory proteins, growth factors, and apoptosis inhibitors, while MAPK signaling stimulates cell division and survival. The combined effects of CagA and LMP proteins on these pathways enhance cellular resistance to stress, promote disruption of cell cycle control, and create a microenvironment favorable for malignant transformation. These mechanisms are key in carcinogenesis, especially in *H. pylori* and EBV coinfection [36, 37]. The CagA oncoprotein produced by virulent strains of *Helicobacter pylori* is capable of causing aberrant activation of the WNT/β-catenin signaling pathway, one of the key regulators of cell proliferation, differentiation, and embryonic development. Under normal conditions, the WNT pathway is strictly controlled and ensures the maintenance of cellular homeostasis, but when exposed to CagA, this balance is disrupted. CagA interferes with the regulation of the stability of β-catenin, one of the central components of WNT signaling, promoting its accumulation in the cytoplasm and subsequent translocation to the nucleus, where it activates the transcription of proto-oncogenes such as c-MYC and cyclin D1. This leads to increased cell proliferation, suppression of apoptosis, and increased cell survival, processes directly associated with oncogenesis. Thus, aberrant activation of the WNT pathway by CagA is an important link in the pathogenesis of *H. pylori*-associated gastric cancer [38]. Activation of the WNT/β-catenin signaling pathway has far-reaching consequences at the molecular level, including the activation of downstream transcription factors such as CDX1. This gene has been shown [39] to play a key role in the reprogramming of mature epithelial cells of the gastric mucosa. Under pathological stimulation, CDX1 promotes the loss of the differentiated phenotype of cells and the acquisition of features characteristic of pluripotent stem cells. CDX1 activates important transcriptional regulators such as SALL4 and KLF5 [40], which are involved in maintaining stemness, enhancing cell proliferation, and self-renewal capacity. These processes underlie cellular plasticity and can promote metaplastic and neoplastic transformations of the epithelium, especially in the context of chronic inflammation caused by *H. pylori* or coinfection with EBV. Thus, WNT-mediated reprogramming via the CDX1–SALL4–KLF5 axis is considered an important link in the pathogenesis of precancerous changes and carcinogenesis in the stomach. Activation of the CDX1–SALL4–KLF5 axis not only promotes the loss of epithelial cells' specific phenotype but also directs their differentiation toward the intestinal type. This process underlies the formation of intestinal metaplasia, a precancerous condition in which the gastric epithelium acquires morphological and functional features of the intestinal epithelium. CDX1, along with its paralog CDX2, is actively involved in the expression of intestinal markers, including MUC2, villin, and sucrase-isomaltase, which reflects a profound reorganization of cellular differentiation. Against the background of chronic inflammation induced by *H. pylori* and possibly aggravated by coinfection with EBV, epithelial cells subjected to such reprogramming become vulnerable to additional mutational and epigenetic changes. Gradual accumulation of such changes can lead to the transition from metaplasia to dysplasia and then to gastric adenocarcinoma, especially of the intestinal type. Thus, the WNT signaling pathway, activated in particular by the CagA oncoprotein, triggers a cascade of molecular events centered on stemness factors and cell identity regulators that promote malignant transformation of the epithelium. The interaction of this pathway with viral and bacterial oncogenes makes it an important target for further research and potential therapeutic strategies.

Data from another study also confirm that both Epstein-Barr virus (EBV) and *Helicobacter pylori* are capable of inducing transformation of the gastric epithelium and directly participating in carcinogenesis. Both infections lead to activation of signaling pathways that disrupt cellular differentiation, stimulate proliferation, and suppress apoptosis, which creates favorable conditions for malignant transformation. The combined effect of viral and bacterial factors, such as EBV LMP1/2 and *H. pylori* CagA, leads to profound molecular and epigenetic reorganization of gastric cells. These changes contribute to the accumulation of genetic damage, disruption of cellular control, and the formation of a tumor phenotype, which emphasizes the importance of coinfection in the pathogenesis of gastric cancer [20]. Both pathogens, *Helicobacter pylori* and Epstein-Barr virus (EBV), are able to induce similar molecular signaling cascades that converge on the activation of transforming factors in gastric epithelial cells. One of the key pathways involved in this process is the β-catenin/TCF-4 signaling pathway. Under the action of the bacterial oncoprotein CagA and viral proteins of EBV, β-catenin is stabilized in the cytoplasm and translocated to the nucleus, where it interacts with the transcription factor TCF-4. This complex activates the expression of proto-oncogenes, such as c-MYC, cyclin D1, and CDX1, which promotes cellular proliferation, suppression of apoptosis, and impairment of differentiation. In conditions of chronic inflammation and coinfection, such an effect increases the risk of malignant transformation of the gastric epithelium, accelerating progression from precancerous conditions to adenocarcinoma. Thus, the β-catenin/TCF-4 signaling pathway represents a crossroad between the pathogenic effects of EBV and *H. pylori* in the development of gastric cancer [25, 41]. Another study found a significant association between Epstein-Barr virus (EBV) and *Helicobacter pylori* positivity and demonstrated marked immune cell infiltration of precancerous areas of the gastric mucosa. Coinfected patients had a high degree of lymphocytic and macrophage infiltration in areas of intestinal metaplasia and dysplasia, which was accompanied by activation of the innate and adaptive immune response. Coinfection leads to the activation of $CD4^+$ and $CD8^+$ T-lymphocytes, which are capable of recognizing both viral and bacterial antigens. This is accompanied by increased expression of pro-inflammatory cytokines such as IFN-γ, TNF-α, IL-1β, IL-6, and IL-8, which enhances inflammation and promotes the recruitment of additional immune cells. Activated macrophages, including the M1 type, secrete inflammatory mediators and molecules that induce oxidative stress, which leads to damage to DNA and the epithelial barrier. In addition, chronic inflammation is accompanied by a violation of the regulation of the Treg/Th17 balance, which can contribute to the long-term persistence of infection and maintenance of the tumor microenvironment. Such a combined effect of the virus and bacteria not only enhances the immunopathological response but also creates conditions for the progression of precancerous changes toward malignant transformation [20]. A study by Szkaradkiewicz et al. demonstrated that the expression of the antiapoptotic protein Bcl-2 was significantly higher in tissues of patients with breast cancer associated with coinfection with Epstein-Barr virus (EBV) and *Helicobacter pylori*. These data suggest that excessive expression of Bcl-2 may be a consequence of the synergistic effect of both pathogens. Since Bcl-2 plays a key role in suppressing programmed cell death and promotes the survival of transformed cells, its increased expression during coinfection may provide an additional advantage to tumor cells, resistance to immune surveillance, and progression of the malignant process. Thus, coinfection with EBV and *H. pylori* can not only enhance inflammatory and proliferative signals but also block apoptosis, which is an important mechanism of carcinogenesis, potentially not limited to the stomach but also to other epithelial tissues, including the mammary gland [42]. Several studies have also shown that protocadherin 10 (PCDH10), a calcium-dependent cell adhesion molecule, plays a tumor suppressor role in gastric epithelial cells. Under normal conditions, PCDH10 is involved in maintaining cell-cell contacts and suppressing uncontrolled proliferation. However, in gastric cancer, especially that associated with *Helicobacter pylori* and Epstein-Barr virus (EBV), hypermethylation of the PCDH10 gene promoter region is observed, which leads to its transcriptional inactivation. Epigenetic suppression of PCDH10 expression disrupts cell-cell connections, promotes loss of epithelial polarity, and facilitates invasive growth of tumor cells. Coinfection with EBV and *H. pylori* may enhance this process due to additional stimulation of inflammatory and signaling cascades involved in DNA methylation. Thus, PCDH10 inactivation through hypermethylation represents one of the key molecular mechanisms by which coinfection promotes the development and progression of gastric malignancies [43–45]. The chromatin remodeling complex SWI/SNF, which is frequently disrupted in gastric cancer (GC), has also been found in association with both Epstein-Barr virus (EBV) and *Helicobacter pylori* infection. This multiprotein complex plays a key role in regulating gene expression by altering chromatin structure and providing access to DNA for transcription factors. Dysfunction of SWI/SNF components such as ARID1A, SMARCA4, and SMARCB1 impairs cellular differentiation, proliferation control, and DNA repair, creating conditions favorable for neoplastic transformation. Both EBV and *H. pylori* have been associated with epigenetic alterations, including chromatin remodeling, and appear to be able to directly or indirectly affect the function of the SWI/SNF complex. For example, expression of viral oncogenes (such as LMP1) and bacterial factors (including CagA) can activate signaling pathways and induce methylation of genes encoding SWI/SNF components. These changes may contribute to the loss of tumor suppression and increased cellular plasticity, making the remodeling complex an important target in the pathogenesis of coinfection-associated gastric cancer [46].

A recent study has shown that the host protein SHP-1 (Src-homology region 2 domain-containing phosphatase-1) is able to interact with the *Helicobacter pylori* oncoprotein CagA, dephosphorylating it and thereby suppressing the oncogenic activity of CagA. This function of SHP-1 is an important protective mechanism that limits the carcinogenic effects of bacterial infection. However, during coinfection with the Epstein-Barr virus (EBV), hypermethylation of the SHP-1 gene promoter occurs, which leads to a decrease in its expression and a loss of dephosphorylation activity toward CagA. As a result, CagA remains in a phosphorylated active form, which enhances its ability to activate signaling pathways associated with cell proliferation, survival, and oncogenesis [47]. In addition, the same study found that EBV and *H. pylori* coinfection was significantly more common in patients with peptic ulcer disease compared to patients with gastroesophageal reflux disease (GERD) or functional dyspepsia [48]. These data suggest a possible link between coinfection and a more aggressive course of upper gastrointestinal diseases, emphasizing the importance of a comprehensive assessment of viral-bacterial interactions in the diagnosis and treatment of such patients. A number of studies indicate that patients infected with *Helicobacter pylori* are more likely to have elevated IgG titers to the Epstein-Barr virus (EBV), which may reflect increased viral activity and more pronounced immune responses from the body [48]. This suggests that *H. pylori* may indirectly promote reactivation of latent EBV and increase its DNA load, possibly through its effects on the inflammatory microenvironment and immunomodulatory pathways. However, there is evidence that *H. pylori* may also play the opposite role. For example, some studies have shown that the bacterium suppresses the expression of TGF-β, a key cytokine that promotes the transition of EBV to the lytic phase [49]. Thus, TGF-β inhibition may limit lytic reactivation of the virus, thereby reducing its carcinogenic potential and theoretically acting as a modulator of viral activity. These contradictory results highlight the complexity of the interaction between *H. pylori* and EBV. It remains unclear under what conditions their coexistence leads to synergy that enhances carcinogenesis and under what conditions they lead to mutual suppression. Therefore, additional studies are needed to elucidate the molecular and immunological mechanisms of their interaction, which will allow a more accurate assessment of the pathogenic role of each of these agents in the development of gastric diseases, including cancer.

11. CMV and *H. pylori*: From simple inflammation to gastric cancer

Cytomegalovirus (CMV), a member of the Herpesviridae family and β-herpesvirinae subfamily, is considered the largest virus infecting humans due to its 235-kilobase double-stranded deoxyribonucleic acid (DNA) genome. Primary CMV infection is usually asymptomatic in immunocompetent individuals but can be a serious clinical problem in immunocompromised patients, including those with HIV infection, after organ transplantation, or against the background of long-term immunosuppression. In these patients, the infection often manifests as severe symptomatic disease. In individuals with preserved immune function, CMV usually becomes latent and may remain inactive throughout life. However, in certain clinical settings, viral reactivation is possible, which is especially relevant in severe inflammatory conditions such as acute respiratory distress syndrome (ARDS). According to recent studies, CMV reactivation is detected in approximately 30% of immunocompetent patients with ARDS and is associated with increased mortality, which emphasizes the potential clinical significance of latent infection even in individuals without severe immunodeficiency. The gastrointestinal tract is one of the main targets for invasive CMV infection. The colon and stomach are most often affected, where the virus causes inflammatory changes, ulceration, and disruption of the mucosal integrity. These manifestations can mimic or accompany other gastrointestinal diseases, including inflammatory bowel disease and peptic ulcer disease, which complicates diagnosis. It is important to note that almost the entire adult population of the globe at some point encounters CMV infection, most often in an asymptomatic form. However, its possible reactivation during systemic inflammation or severe stress of the body makes CMV an important object of observation not only in immunocompromised patients but also in immunocompetent patients with severe critical conditions [50].

Human herpesvirus 5 (HHV-5), better known as cytomegalovirus (CMV), is a widespread member of the Herpesviridae family, infecting between 40 and 70% of the population worldwide [51, 52]. Following primary infection, CMV enters a lifelong latency state, predominantly localizing in myeloid cells such as monocytes and their precursors. This mechanism allows the virus to effectively evade immune surveillance without causing symptoms in most immunocompetent hosts. However, under conditions of immunosuppression, either pharmacological (e.g., during organ transplantation) or natural (during aging or severe systemic diseases), the virus can reactivate, causing clinically significant lesions, particularly in target organs such as the gastrointestinal tract, lungs, and central nervous system. Although *Helicobacter pylori* has traditionally occupied a central place in research on the pathogenesis of gastrointestinal diseases, the impact of coinfections with other microbes, including herpes viruses, remains poorly understood. Meanwhile, CMV, as one of the most common herpesvirus infections, deserves special attention given its potential ability to modify the immune responses of the gastric and intestinal mucosa, as well as affect the course of *H. pylori*-associated diseases. Thus, further studies are needed to identify the interactions between *H. pylori* and CMV, their possible synergism or antagonism, as well as the impact on inflammation, ulceration, and tumor transformation in the gastrointestinal tract.

11.1 CMV reactivation in the gastrointestinal tract and the impact on the immune microenvironment

In conditions of immune imbalance or systemic inflammation, CMV is able to exit the latent state and reactivate, which is especially often observed in the mucous membrane of the gastrointestinal tract. The colon and stomach are among the main targets for the invasive form of the disease. Reactivation is accompanied by viral replication in epithelial cells and cells of the lamina propria of the mucosa, which leads to a cytopathic effect, inflammation, and ulceration. The immune microenvironment created by CMV in the gastrointestinal tract is characterized by:

- Active infiltration of T-lymphocytes (mainly $CD8^{+}$), aimed at controlling the virus, which is accompanied by a pronounced inflammatory response;
- Increased production of proinflammatory cytokines, including TNF-α, IFN-γ, IL-6, and IL-1β, which aggravate local tissue damage;
- Activation of macrophages and dendritic cells that promote antigen presentation and maintain chronic inflammation;
- Increased expression of apoptosis and oxidative stress molecules that lead to impaired mucosal regeneration;
- Decreased regulatory T cells (Treg) and an imbalance between Th1/Th17 responses, which can enhance autoaggression.

The accumulation of such immunological changes can not only complicate the healing of the mucous membrane but also modify the course of other infections, including *Helicobacter pylori*. It is assumed that CMV reactivation in the stomach against the background of *H. pylori* persistence can enhance the inflammatory background, disrupt the regulation of cellular proliferation and apoptosis, and create conditions for dysplastic changes and malignant transformation of the epithelium. Some experimental data also indicate that cytomegalovirus is able to suppress the expression of key immunoregulators, including TGF-β and IL-10, as well as interfere with the NF-κB and STAT3 signaling pathways, which further contributes to the chronicity of inflammation and disruption of immune homeostasis in the gastric mucosa.

Quite an interesting study was published by Zamani et al. [53]. This study was conducted in Iraq (January–March 2022). The study focused on 90 patients with suspected *H. pylori* infection, with clinical symptoms of abdominal pain, flatulence (bloating), unexplained loss of appetite, and nausea. The authors enrolled these patients in the study, with initial randomization into two groups: *H. pylori* IgG-positive (positive group) and *H. pylori* IgG-negative (negative group). Screening serological tests based on the determination of the presence of specific IgG in venous blood samples were used to detect antibodies to *Helicobacter pylori*. The level of IgG antibodies to cytomegalovirus (CMV) was determined by enzyme-linked immunosorbent assay (ELISA) using the automated Mini VIDAS system (bioMérieux, France). This semiquantitative test allows for a high sensitivity and specificity in assessing the presence and level of circulating antibodies indicative of current or past infection. Combined serologic testing for *H. pylori* and CMV was used to analyze potential coinfection and to study the relationship between viral and bacterial load in the examined patients. The study found that the level of IgG antibodies to cytomegalovirus (CMV) significantly differed between the *Helicobacter pylori*-negative and -positive groups. In individuals not infected with *H. pylori*, the average titer of antibodies to CMV was 52.41 ± 24.107, while in those infected, it was significantly higher—70.39 ± 29.048 (P = 0.002). Moreover, a statistically significant positive correlation was found between the serostatus for *H. pylori* and the level of antibodies to CMV (r = 0.323, P = 0.003), which indicates a possible relationship between the presence of a bacterial infection and an increased viral load or immune activation in relation to CMV.

Analysis by gender showed that men were infected with *H. pylori* more often than women—63.16 versus 38.5%, respectively. Statistical analysis demonstrated that male gender can be considered a risk factor for *H. pylori* infection, with an odds ratio (OR) of 2.74 (95% confidence interval: 1.15–6.5; P = 0.032). At the same time, CMV antibody titers did not show significant differences between men and women: in men, the mean value was 61.00 ± 23.85, and in women, 61.35 ± 30.88 (P > 0.05).

In conclusion, the obtained results allowed the authors to make several important findings.

First, the above study found that men (63.16%) were significantly more likely to be infected with *H. pylori* than women (38.5%), which allows us to consider male gender as an independent risk factor for infection. The odds ratio (OR) calculation showed a statistically significant association: OR = 2.74 (95% confidence interval: 1.15–6.5; P = 0.032). These results are consistent with global data, according to which the *H. pylori* infection rate among men is on average 46.3%, while in women it is 42.7% [53]. These differences may be due to both behavioral and epidemiological factors, as well as possible gender differences in immune response and susceptibility to bacterial colonization. Given the parallel prevalence of chronic CMV infection, further studies are needed to examine the impact of gender and viral-bacterial interactions on the risk and course of diseases associated with these pathogens.

Second, a moderate positive correlation was found between *H. pylori* infection and cytomegalovirus (CMV) antibody levels (r = 0.323; P = 0.003), indicating a possible interaction between these two pathogens. The widespread global distribution of *Helicobacter pylori* and the high incidence of chronic cytomegalovirus (CMV) infection in the population indicate a potentially significant inflammatory interaction between two persistent pathogens, which deserves close attention. These infections, despite differences in transmission mechanisms and pathogenesis, may overlap in the same mucosal environment, especially in the gastrointestinal tract, promoting chronic inflammation and immune imbalance. However, the question of causality between them remains open: does *H. pylori* promote reactivation of latent CMV infection by causing chronic inflammation and mucosal immunosuppression, or does CMV infection modulate the immune response, increasing susceptibility to *H. pylori*? Further prospective, mechanistic, and multicenter studies are needed to definitively establish the mechanisms of such interaction.

Third, the analysis of the data obtained in the study showed that there were no significant differences in CMV antibody titers between the age groups, with the exception of the comparison of the 40–61- and 61–87-year-old groups, where a tendency toward an increase in titers was recorded in the older age category. However, the overall statistical significance of the differences by age did not reach the established threshold (P = 0.11), which may indicate a moderate but not reliable increase in the CMV viral load with age. As for *Helicobacter pylori* infection, there were no statistically significant age differences in the infection rates in the study sample (P = 0.51), indicating a uniform distribution of the infection among different age groups. These data suggest that *H. pylori* is a stable and persistent infection independent of age in middle and old age. Results of other studies have shown that the prevalence of *Helicobacter pylori* and cytomegalovirus (CMV) infection varies significantly depending on the geographic region and socioeconomic conditions. In particular, both pathogens show a significantly higher prevalence in low- and middle-income countries compared to industrialized regions. This phenomenon has traditionally been attributed to factors such as poor sanitation, limited access to clean water, overcrowding, and inadequate health infrastructure. Such differences have been previously reviewed in detail in a number of epidemiological studies, which emphasize the importance of socioeconomic determinants in the spread of chronic infections. These data highlight the need to take into account regional and social factors when planning screening, prevention, and treatment programs for *H. pylori* and CMV infections [54–56]. According to epidemiological data, the prevalence of *Helicobacter pylori* in the European population ranged from 20 to 40% 10 years ago, depending on the country, age of the subjects, and socioeconomic conditions. Lower infection rates were observed in Northern and Western Europe, while infection rates remained higher in Eastern and Southern Europe. This decrease in prevalence in some regions is associated with improved sanitary and hygienic conditions, higher living standards, availability of antibiotics, and early detection and eradication programs. However, *H. pylori* continues to be an important clinical problem in a number of countries with limited resources, as well as among migrant and vulnerable populations, even in developed countries [57]. In a cross-sectional study conducted in the United States, the prevalence of *Helicobacter pylori* infection among children under 3 years of age was 25.4%, indicating the possibility of very early infection, probably through intrafamilial or vertical transmission. These results highlight the importance of early life as a “critical window” for initial infection and subsequent persistence of infection [58]. In Japan, the prevalence of *Helicobacter pylori* shows marked cohort differences. According to published data, among individuals born before the 1950s, the infection rate reached almost 90%, reflecting the historically high incidence of disease associated with living conditions and hygiene in the postwar period. However, since the end of the twentieth century, there has been a gradual and steady decline in the prevalence of infection, with the prevalence falling to less than 2% among cohorts born after 2000. This epidemiological shift has key public health implications, particularly in the context of Japan, which has traditionally had a high incidence of gastric cancer, which is closely associated with persistent *H. pylori* infection. Given the well-documented association between *H. pylori* and the development of gastritis, intestinal metaplasia, and gastric adenocarcinoma, the decline in infection rates in younger generations may herald a significant reduction in cancer incidence in the coming decades. This trend highlights the importance of early detection and eradication programs as an effective measure for the primary prevention of gastric cancer [59]. However, in some regions of the world, the prevalence of *Helicobacter pylori* infection remains extremely high. In particular, according to epidemiological studies, the prevalence of infection reaches up to 80% among the adult population in the

Eastern Mediterranean countries. These rates reflect high endemicity and are due to a number of factors, including poor sanitation, high population density, limited access to health care and diagnostics, and frequent intrafamilial transmission of the pathogen. The high incidence of infection in this region requires special attention in public health programs aimed at the control and eradication of *H. pylori*, especially given its association with gastritis, peptic ulcer disease, and gastric cancer [60].

According to previous studies, the population of the southwestern region of Mexico demonstrates a higher probability of coinfection with several pathogens, including *Helicobacter pylori*, Epstein-Barr virus (EBV), and cytomegalovirus (CMV). All these infectious agents are closely associated with gastric carcinogenesis and play an important role in the development of chronic inflammation of the mucosa. A particularly high frequency of EBV and CMV coinfections was noted among patients with gastritis and gastric cancer. A significant proportion of these patients also had concomitant coinfection with *H. pylori* in EBV/*H. pylori* or CMV/*H. pylori* combinations, indicating the potential for synergistic interaction of pathogens in the formation of a stable inflammatory background and subsequent oncogenic process. Importantly, Epstein-Barr virus is detected in malignant gastric tumors regardless of the histological type of neoplasm, indicating its universal role in carcinogenesis. However, despite the identified associations, mechanistic questions remain open. In particular, it is unclear whether *H. pylori* promotes the initiation of the lytic phase of EBV, which may lead to reactivation of latent viral infection. Similarly, there is no clear data on whether *H. pylori* can play a role in the reactivation of latent CMV, which in turn could influence the progression of inflammatory and proliferative changes in the gastric mucosa. To clarify these aspects, additional experimental and clinical studies aimed at understanding the relationship between bacterial and viral agents in the context of gastroduodenal diseases and gastric cancer are needed [61].

Another study investigated the relationship between gastrointestinal cancer (GI) and cytomegalovirus (CMV) and *Helicobacter pylori* coinfection. Polymerase chain reaction (PCR) was used to analyze paired gastric tumor and surrounding peritumoral tissue samples from 134 patients, including 98 men and 36 women. The results showed that *H. pylori* infection was detected in 74 patients (55.2%), and CMV infection was detected in 58 patients (43.3%). Coinfection with both pathogens was detected in 34 patients (25.4%). Risk factor analysis demonstrated that *H. pylori* infection was independently associated with progressive lymphatic metastasis in tumor processes in both univariate and multivariate analyses ($P = 0.007$; odds ratio $OR = 3.51$). Interestingly, tumors coinfected with *H. pylori* and CMV showed a reduced propensity for lymphatic metastasis compared to tumors infected with *H. pylori* alone. This unexpected observation suggests a possible interaction between CMV and *H. pylori* that may influence the metastatic process. This finding requires further studies to clarify the molecular and immunological mechanisms of interaction between these pathogens, as well as their potential role in regulating lymphatic dissemination in gastrointestinal cancer [62].

Menetrier disease associated with coinfection with cytomegalovirus (CMV) and *Helicobacter pylori* is an extremely rare clinical case that was documented in a patient from Asia. It is interesting to note that all known cases of coinfection, to our knowledge, were described mainly in pediatric practice in Asian countries. This circumstance may be important for a deep understanding of the etiology, pathogenesis, and progression of this disease. Such regional specificity probably reflects the peculiarities of the epidemiology and pathogenesis of CMV and *H. pylori* in East Asia, where, in contrast to Europe and Western countries, a high prevalence of these infections remains, especially among the child population and in developing regions. High morbidity and widespread distribution of both pathogens create conditions for more frequent cases of coinfection, which may affect the clinical picture and severity of the disease. Thus, cases of Menetrier disease due to CMV and *H. pylori* coinfection may not be as rare in these regions as expected and require closer attention in pediatric gastroenterology and infectious pathology. Additional clinical and epidemiological studies are needed to identify risk factors and develop optimal diagnostic and therapeutic strategies [63, 64].

In immunocompromised patients, such as those with a history of allotransplantation, cancer, acquired immunodeficiency syndrome (AIDS), or those receiving long-term immunosuppressive therapy, primary cytomegalovirus (CMV) infection may present with a severe clinical course. In such cases, multiorgan involvement is observed, including the gastrointestinal tract and central nervous system. In contrast, in immunocompetent individuals, CMV infection usually has a milder course: patients often remain asymptomatic, and the disease may not be diagnosed at all. However, in some cases, CMV infection may present with clinical features similar to a viral infection or a syndrome resembling infectious mononucleosis [65–67].

Invasive gastrointestinal tract disease in primary cytomegalovirus (CMV) infection is quite rare, and only a few such cases have been described in the scientific literature [68, 69]. After resolution of the primary infection, CMV can persist in the host body for many years. This is possible due to the presence of many molecules in the virus that help evade the immune response, which allows CMV to maintain a latent state mainly in the myeloid and stem cells of the host throughout life [51, 70]. In immunocompromised individuals, the risk of CMV reactivation increases significantly, which is due to a decrease in the effectiveness of immune control over the virus [71, 72]. In individuals with preserved immune status, despite relative resistance to severe infections, there are factors that can provoke reactivation of latent cytomegalovirus (CMV). These factors include chronic diseases, such as liver cirrhosis, as well as acute stress conditions—severe injuries, burns, shock, and other significant damage to the body. These conditions lead to a weakening of immune control, which facilitates the exit of the virus from the latent state and the development of reactivation. Reactivated CMV infection in immunocompetent patients may manifest as severe systemic morbidity, involving multiple organs and systems. The most common clinical manifestations are neurological disorders (including encephalitis and polyneuritis), hematological abnormalities (cytopenia and bone marrow dysfunction), cardiovascular system damage (myocarditis), ophthalmological complications (including chorioretinitis), and gastrointestinal tract damage. It should be noted separately that invasive gastric damage in primary CMV infection in immunocompetent individuals is an extremely rare phenomenon and has been documented only in isolated cases. However, it is during virus reactivation in this group of patients that these lesions occur much more often. In such situations, CMV can cause ulcerative changes, inflammatory processes, and other morphological damage to the gastric mucosa, which requires increased attention from clinicians for timely diagnosis and treatment. Thus, even in patients with normal immune status, the risk of CMV reactivation should be taken into account in the presence of predisposing factors and clinical manifestations, which helps prevent severe complications and improve the prognosis of the disease [73, 74].

A study by Hulo P. and colleagues described a rare case of a 42-year-old immunocompetent male patient who complained of acute, increasing pain in the umbilical region [74]. During endoscopic examination, inflammation of the gastric mucosa was detected, which allowed the diagnosis of acute gastritis caused by cytomegalovirus (CMV) infection. In addition, histological analysis of gastric biopsy samples also revealed signs of chronic active gastritis associated with the presence of *Helicobacter pylori*. The diagnosis was based on the results of histopathological examination, confirming inflammatory changes characteristic of CMV infection, as well as morphological signs typical of gastritis associated with *H. pylori*. The endoscopic and pathomorphological examination data are presented in **Figures 4–6** [74].

This case illustrates that even in patients with normal immune status, several infectious agents may be present simultaneously, which requires careful diagnostics and an individualized approach to treatment [74]. In immunocompromised patients, primary cytomegalovirus (CMV) infection is usually accompanied by severe symptoms and a severe clinical course. At the same time, in people with normal immunity, the infection is often asymptomatic or remains latent for many years. If CMV infection manifests itself with clinically significant symptoms in immunocompetent patients, it most often resembles a common viral disease or a syndrome similar to infectious mononucleosis. The clinical picture is nonspecific and includes such signs as fever, discomfort or pain in the upper abdomen (epigastric region), loss of appetite, nausea, vomiting, bowel disorders in the form of diarrhea or constipation, as well as the appearance of a skin rash. These symptoms require careful examination and differentiation from other diseases of the gastrointestinal tract in order to promptly identify CMV infection and prescribe adequate treatment [2, 75, 76].

In immunocompetent individuals, primary cytomegalovirus (CMV) infection rarely results in invasive disease. In most cases, clinically significant lesions in this group of patients are due to reactivation of latent infection. The gastrointestinal tract is of greatest clinical significance, followed by involvement of the hematopoietic system and the central nervous system. Less common are lesions of the eye, liver, and respiratory system [77]. Among the gastrointestinal tract sites, the colon and stomach are most frequently involved. However, the molecular and cellular mechanisms by which CMV infects the gastric mucosa are not fully understood. One hypothesis suggests that viral activation results in transiently elevated levels of transforming growth factor-α (TGF-α). This factor is able to interact with epidermal growth factor receptors (EGFRs) localized on the surface of cells in the gastric mucosa. Activation of these receptors stimulates cellular proliferation, increased mucus secretion, and the development of hypertrophic gastropathy. Moreover, it is believed that EGFR

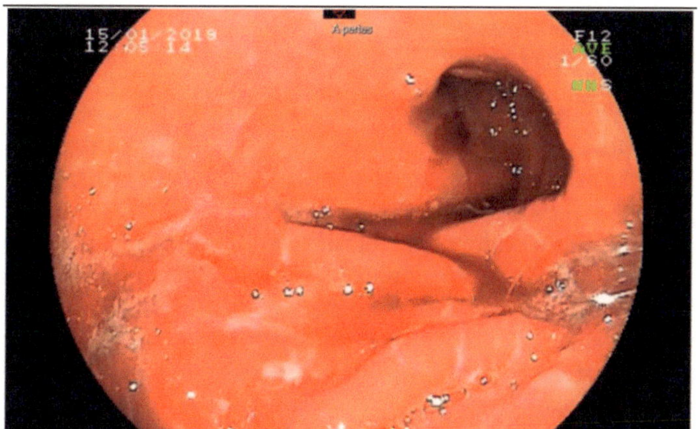

Figure 4.
Endoscopic images of the gastric fundus (left), cardia (right), and body of the stomach (right) showing severe erosive gastritis with prominent erythematous and edematous gastric folds (adapted from Hulo et al. [74]).

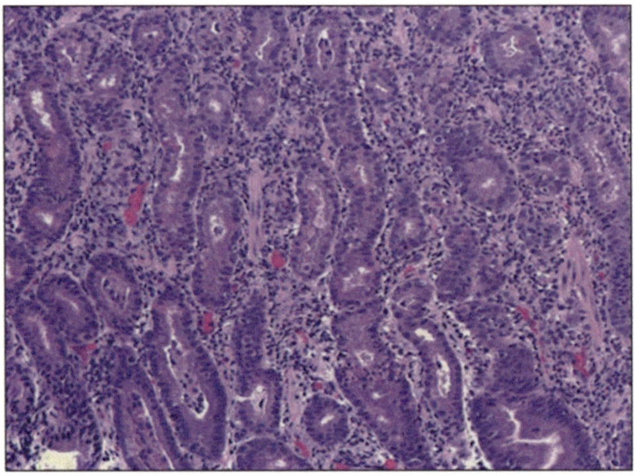

Figure 5.
Histopathological findings of gastric biopsy: gastric mucosal fragments from the antrum showing significant infiltration of neutrophils and lymphocytes into the lamina propria (adapted from Hulo et al. [74]).

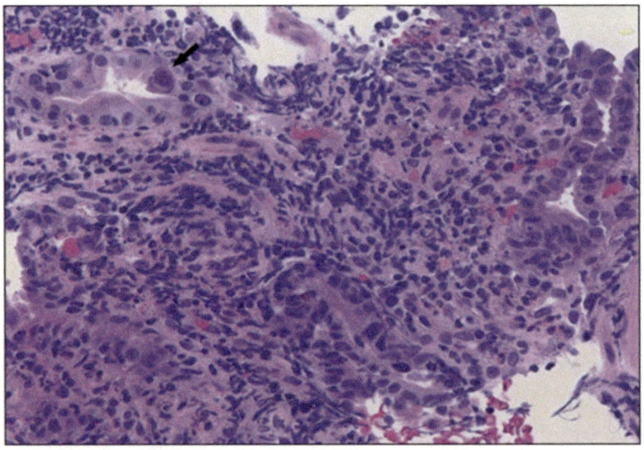

Figure 6.
Histopathological findings of gastric biopsy: fragments of the gastric antral mucosa containing cytomegalovirus inclusions (adapted from Hulo et al. [74]).

activation may contribute to increased vascular permeability associated with cytomegalovirus vasculitis, which in turn leads to mucosal protein leakage and may manifest clinically as protein-losing gastroenteropathy [63, 78, 79].

Cytomegalovirus infection of the gastrointestinal tract may be accompanied by a wide range of clinical and endoscopic manifestations, often nonspecific and variable in their morphology. The endoscopic picture varies from minor changes, such as "spotted areas" of erythema, exudate deposits, or superficial microerosions, to more pronounced lesions—pronounced edema of the mucous membrane, deep round ulcers, and even formations that imitate tumors (pseudotumors) [80, 81]. One of the difficulties in diagnosis is the lack of specificity of the endoscopic picture: gastric ulcers caused by CMV infection are difficult to distinguish from ulcers caused by *Helicobacter pylori* or the use of nonsteroidal anti-inflammatory drugs (NSAIDs) [82]. In CMV gastritis, the most common findings are mucosal hyperemia, erythematous areas, erosive changes, and ulcers. However, fewer characteristic features have been described in some cases, including inflammatory pseudopolyps, hypertrophy of gastric folds, and diffuse mucosal edema with thickening of gastric rugae [83, 84]. These features emphasize the need for histological examination and verification of the diagnosis using molecular methods (e.g., PCR or immunohistochemistry), especially in patients with unclear gastric complaints and negative results for *H. pylori* and NSAID-associated lesions.

According to a recent case series of 30 patients with confirmed cytomegalovirus (CMV) infection of the upper gastrointestinal tract, both immunocompetent and immunocompromised individuals, it was found that lesions were usually localized within a single anatomical segment. The most frequently involved region was the antrum (antropyloric zone) of the stomach, which may be related to the physiological characteristics of secretion and accumulation of gastric contents in this zone. The second most frequently affected organs were the cardia, then the lower third of the esophagus, and, to a lesser extent, the duodenum. These data emphasize a certain anatomical and topographic predictability of the localization of CMV-induced inflammatory changes in the upper gastrointestinal tract. Given the non-specificity of clinical symptoms, such data are especially important for focused endoscopic diagnostics with targeted biopsy from the indicated areas when CMV gastroduodenitis is suspected [85].

Given the nonspecific nature of endoscopic changes in cytomegalovirus gastritis, diagnosis requires a comprehensive approach based on a combination of clinical presentation, histopathological findings, and laboratory confirmation of viral infection. The main methods for verifying the diagnosis are viral DNA amplification (e.g., PCR) and immunohistochemical detection of viral antigens in tissue sections. From a histological point of view, characteristic features of CMV gastritis are foveolar hyperplasia, mucosal infiltration with lymphocytes and plasma cells (lymphoplasmacytic infiltrate), and the presence of pathognomonic eosinophilic intracellular inclusions known as "owl's eye bodies"—a consequence of viral replication in cells. It should be noted that standard hematoxylin and eosin staining does not always reveal viral inclusions, especially if CMV infects vascular endothelial cells or stromal elements in the submucosal layer under ulcerative defects. In such cases, immunohistochemical methods and molecular diagnostics significantly increase diagnostic sensitivity and specificity [5, 15]. In order to increase diagnostic accuracy in detecting cytomegalovirus (CMV) infection of the gastrointestinal tract, it is advisable to combine endoscopic methods with highly specific laboratory and molecular studies. Due to the fact that the endoscopic picture in CMV gastritis is often nonspecific and can imitate other inflammatory or ulcerative lesions, the isolated use of this method is not enough for reliable diagnosis.

The most informative and sensitive additions to endoscopic examination are:

- quantitative polymerase chain reaction (PCR) for detection and assessment of the viral load of CMV DNA in tissue biopsies or blood;
- DNA *in situ* hybridization, which allows visualization of viral DNA directly in the context of the cellular structure of the tissue;
- immunohistochemical staining aimed at detecting CMV antigens in the gastric mucosa or other affected areas. The integrated use of these methods, especially in combination with clinical and histological assessment, significantly increases diagnostic sensitivity and allows identifying both active and latent forms of infection, which is important for differential diagnosis and choice of therapeutic tactics [86–88].

Despite the fact that, in case of damage to the central nervous system, respiratory system, and visual organ caused by cytomegalovirus (CMV) infection, antiviral therapy is considered justified and recommended [10], to date, there are no unified clinical guidelines regulating the prescription of specific antiviral drugs for CMV gastritis in immunocompetent patients. In individuals with preserved immune status, CMV gastritis is usually characterized by a benign and self-limited course that does not require specific drug intervention. In such cases, preference is given to supportive and symptomatic treatment with monitoring of clinical dynamics [2]. The question of the advisability of prescribing antiviral therapy for CMV infection in immunocompetent patients remains open. Perhaps certain categories of such patients—especially those who demonstrate a severe or protracted course of the disease or have potential hidden risk factors—can receive clinical benefit from etiotropic treatment. However, to date, there is not enough evidence to develop clear clinical recommendations; therefore, further studies are needed to assess the risks and effectiveness of antiviral therapy in this population. Given that gastrointestinal forms of CMV infection predominantly develop in individuals with impaired immune systems, the diagnosis of such lesions in a patient without obvious signs of immunosuppression should prompt a search for hidden pathological conditions. It is important to exclude the presence of oncological diseases, such as lymphomas, autoimmune processes, or other forms of immunodeficiency that could contribute to the development of the disease. In support of this, one observational study found that 4 out of 11 patients with clinically confirmed CMV gastritis, initially considered immunocompetent, were subsequently diagnosed with a malignant tumor. Thus, when diagnosing CMV infection of the gastrointestinal tract in a previously healthy patient, it is advisable to conduct an in-depth examination to exclude latent forms of immunosuppression [19, 89–93].

It seems quite significant that a number of studies indicate a potential contribution of chronic inflammation caused by cytomegalovirus (CMV) infection to the progression of *Helicobacter pylori*-associated gastritis and, as a consequence, to the development of gastric cancer. Thus, according to the study by Moral-Hernández et al., the prevalence of *H. pylori* among patients with chronic gastritis was 48.1%, while CMV infection was detected in 52.8% of cases [94]. Moreover, CMV was detected in 53.1% of gastric carcinoma samples, which may indicate its direct participation in carcinogenesis. Considering that persistent inflammation is recognized as an important oncogenic factor, it becomes likely that CMV can contribute to the development of malignant neoplasms of the stomach both independently and due to a synergistic interaction with *H. pylori*. This assumption is supported by the results of a recent meta-analysis, which established a reliable association between human CMV infection and gastrointestinal tumors [95]. In light of these data, timely detection and treatment of both infections is of particular importance. Missed or unrecognized cases of *H. pylori* and CMV coinfection may pose a significant oncological risk to patients, especially in the presence of chronic gastritis or other precancerous changes in the gastric mucosa.

12. Issues of herpesvirus lesions in patients with *Helicobacter pylori* (results of own research)

Thus, at the beginning of our research, there were already certain statements, in particular:

Statement 1. *H. pylori* infection is accepted as the major etiological factor for gastric cancer. (Level of evidence: 1a Grade of recommendation: A) [96].

This is now established beyond doubt from numerous strands of evidence, including epidemiology, molecular studies, animal studies, and eradication studies in humans, showing a reduced incidence of gastric cancer in those receiving eradication therapy. While Epstein-Barr virus and other rare causes (including hereditary ones) might account for a small proportion of gastric cancers worldwide, it is acknowledged that at least 90% of cancers are related to *H. pylori* infection. The risk of cancer arising from *H. pylori* infection is identical for gastric cancer of both intestinal and diffuse types.

Statement 4. The influence of environmental factors is subordinate to the effect of *H. pylori* infection. (Level of evidence: 2a Grade of recommendation: A) [96].

It is unclear whether the small fraction of cases where *H. pylori* is not detectable is associated with other etiologic factors (e.g., Epstein-Barr virus) or is related to misclassification. Moreover, it is unknown whether cofactors are necessary in all cases or whether infection alone leads to gastric cancer.

Statement 1. *H. pylori* infection is the primary etiological factor for gastric adenocarcinoma, including proximal gastric cancer (PGC). (Agreement 100% Grade A1) [97].

Statement 6. *H. pylori* infection and EBV are independent risk factors of gastric cancer. Whether coinfection of *H. pylori* and EBV is associated with a higher risk of gastric cancer than either one alone remains uncertain. (Agreement 97%, Grade C2) [97].

EBV is associated with gastric lymphoepithelioma-like carcinomas, which have a relatively higher frequency in proximal locations and diffuse histological subtypes. A comprehensive molecular characterization further showed that EBV-associated gastric adenocarcinoma displayed recurrent PIK3CA mutations, extreme DNA hypermethylation, and amplification of JAK2, PD-L1, and PD-L2.

A recent systematic review and meta-analysis of case-control studies showed that the pooled prevalence of EBV was 8.8% in 20,361 patients with gastric cancer. Of the 20 studies with a matched pairs design from 4116 gastric cancer patients, EBV was associated with an 18-fold increased risk of gastric cancer. Some case-control studies showed that coinfection of *H. pylori* and EBV was associated with more severe gastric inflammation and increased risk of gastric cancer. However, evidence from cohort studies or nested case-control studies is lacking on this issue [97].

Invasive gastric carcinoma is preceded by a cascade of precancerous lesions. The first recognized histologic change is active chronic inflammation, which may persist as such: non-atrophic chronic gastritis (no gland loss) or advance to multifocal atrophic gastritis (MAG), the first real step in the precancerous cascade. The following steps are intestinal metaplasia (first "complete" and then "incomplete") and dysplasia, first low grade and then high grade (equivalent to "carcinoma in situ"). The following step is invasive carcinoma.

And of course, the pressing question came to the fore: *Why is stomach cancer increasing?*

After all, it seems that the main recommendations are being followed:

- Routine endoscopy is performed, and *H. pylori* is checked (in 95% of patients)
- *H. pylori*-positive patients receive treatment
- *H. pylori* negative in repeated examinations

Considering the rather high prevalence of *H. pylori* in the world, the role of both *H. pylori* and herpes viruses (in particular EBV) in the malignancy of the stomach and duodenum, the issues of timely and adequate diagnosis of herpes viruses in patients with *H. pylori* remain open and still unresolved from the standpoint of issues: when and from whom to conduct this search.

Aim: to identify the frequency of occurrence of herpes viruses in patients with successful eradication of *H. pylori* but with persistent clinical complaints.

Materials and methods: In the period from December 2019 to August 2021, 560 patients with *H. pylori* (*H. pylori* was detected by the CLO test and by the histological method) were identified, who underwent eradication therapy. In 89 patients (15.9%), despite the positive results of the eradication therapy, clinical complaints persisted (heartburn, epigastric pain, flatulence); this group of patients was re-examined, and endoscopic examination of the stomach and duodenum was performed, with biopsy sampling for pathomorphological examination and diagnosis by polymerase chain reaction for herpes viruses in biopsies (HSV I/II, EBV, CMV, HHV6). Biopsy sites: from stomach (antrum-2 biopsy, corpus-2 biopsy), from duodenum (bulbus-4 biopsy), and from visually altered areas of the mucous membrane of the stomach and duodenum. The distribution of patients is shown in **Figure 7**.

As a result, in 61 patients (68.5%; 34 men, 27 women, age from 19 to 65 years, mean age 35.2 ± 2.4 years), herpes viruses (HSVI/II, EBV, CMV, and HHV6) were found. Distribution of biopsies: from the duodenum in 56 patients (91.8 and 62.9%, respectively) and from the stomach in 5 patients (8.2 and 5.62%, respectively).

As a result, duodenal biopsy specimens revealed HHV6 in 23 cases (41.1 and 37.7%), CMV in 2 cases (3.57 and 3.27%), HSVI+II in 14 cases (25 and 22.9%), and EBV in 14 cases (25 and 22.9%). In gastric biopsies, in 3 cases (60 and 4.92%), HHV6 and in 2 cases (40 and 3.27%), EBV. A description of mono-herpesvirus lesions is presented in **Figure 8**.

Some results of pathomorphological studies of our patients are presented in **Figures 9–11** (from the personal archive data of Dr. J. Musayev).

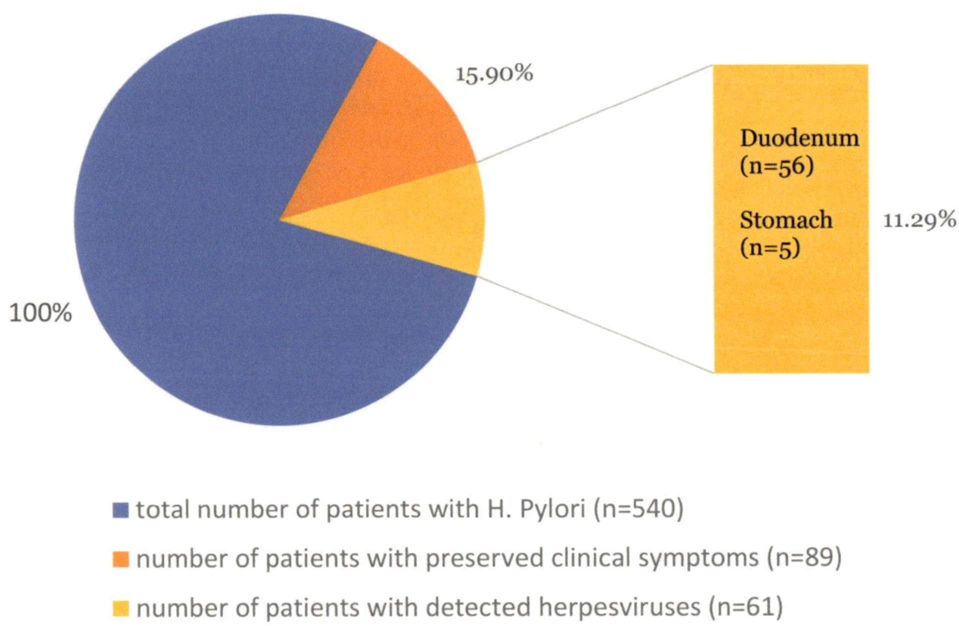

Figure 7.
Distribution of patients.

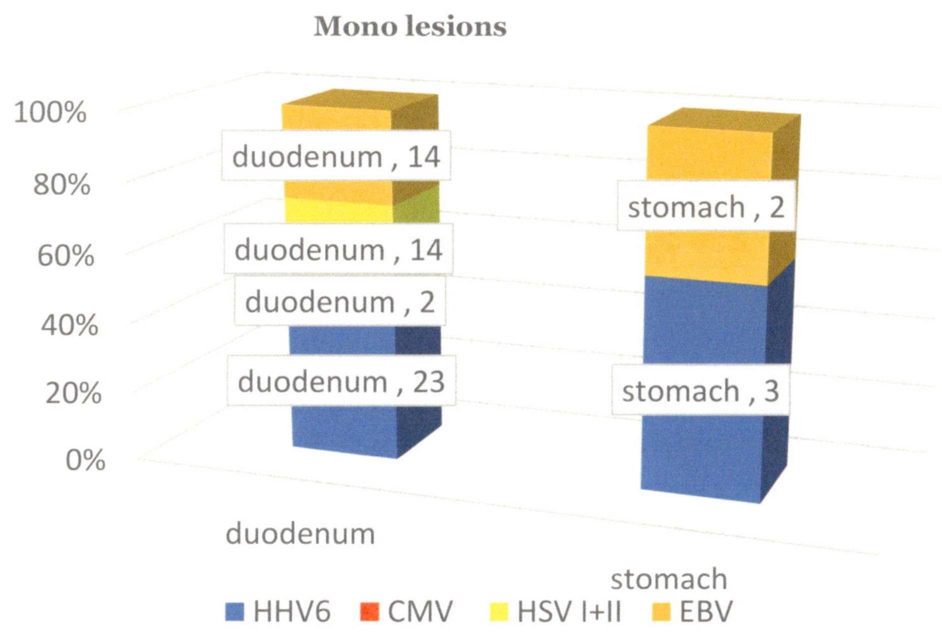

Figure 8.
Mono-herpesvirus lesions of the stomach and duodenum.

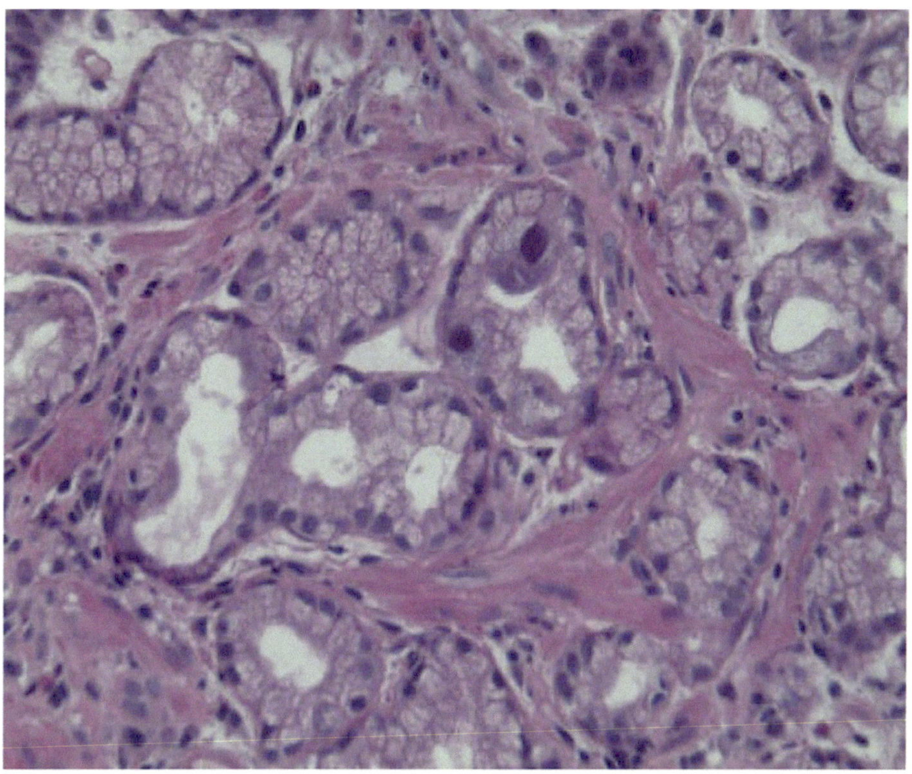

Figure 9.
*CMV+/*H. pylori.

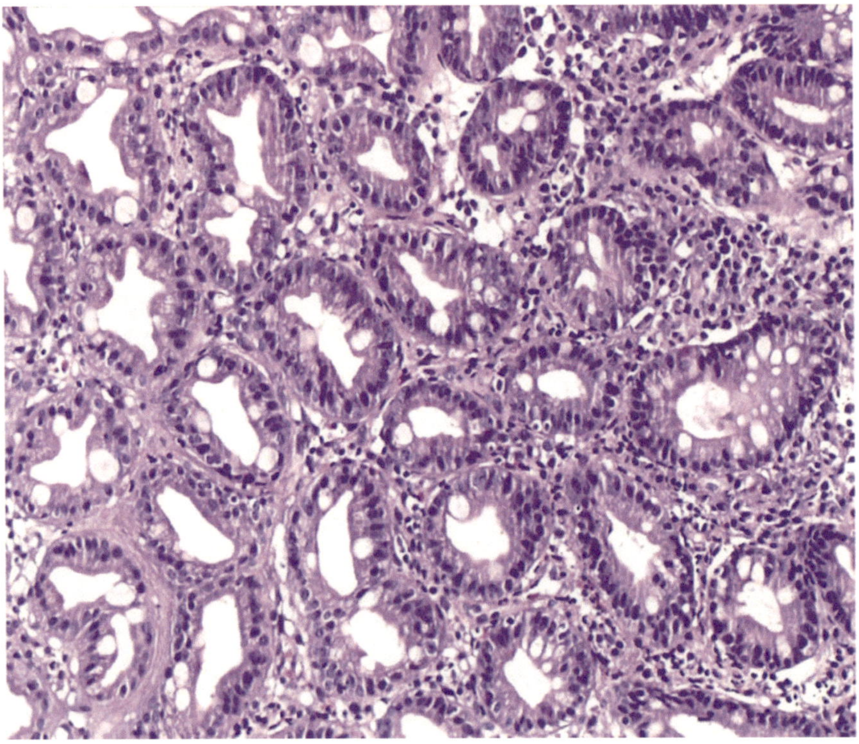

Figure 10.
HHV6+/H. pylori.

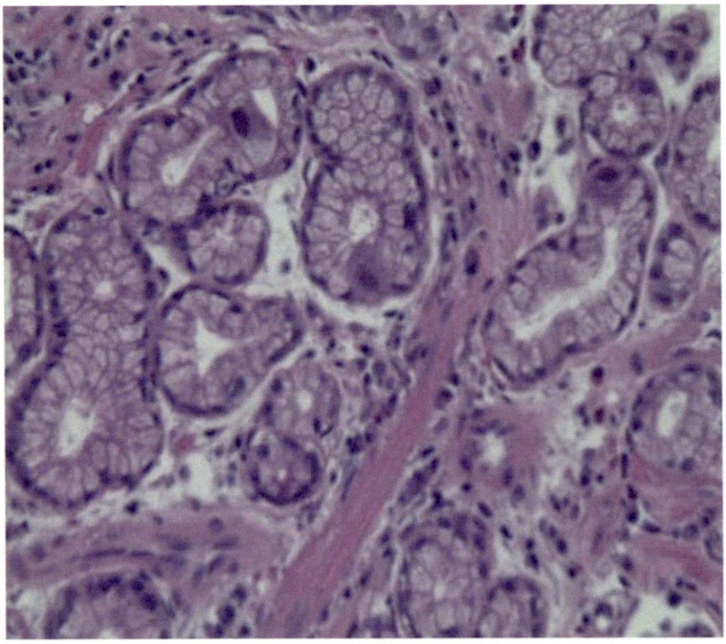

Figure 11.
CMV+/*EBV+*/H. pylori.

Some endoscopic images of this group of patients are presented in **Figures 12–14** (from the archives of Dr. Umud Mahmudov).

The study revealed cases with combined herpes virus lesions of the gastric and duodenal mucosa (**Figure 15**). Thus, the number of combined lesions in the duodenum: HHV6 + EBV in 2 patients (3.57 and 3.27%); HHV6 + CMV in 1 patient (1.78

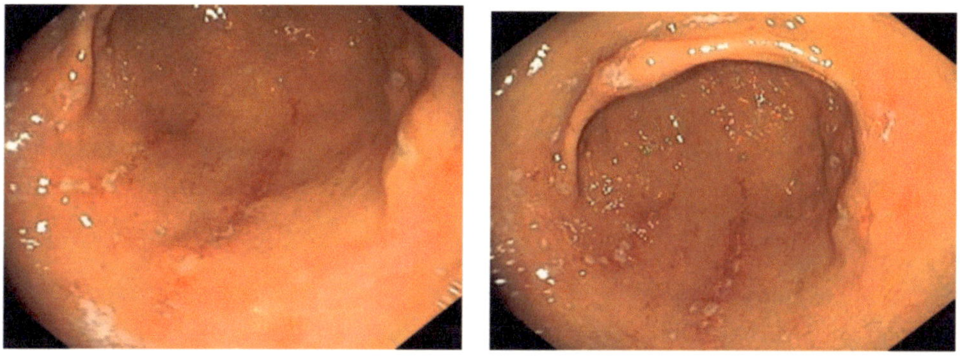

Figure 12.
Stomach: Helicobacter pylori *(positive).*

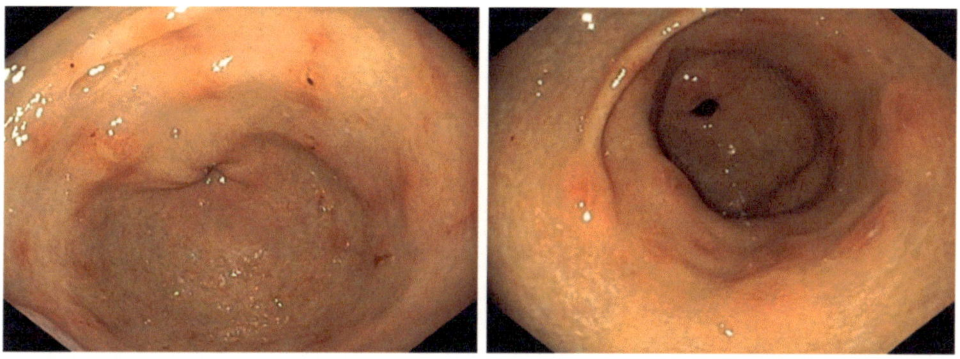

Figure 13.
Stomach: Helicobacter pylori *(negative) and HSV I/II (positive).*

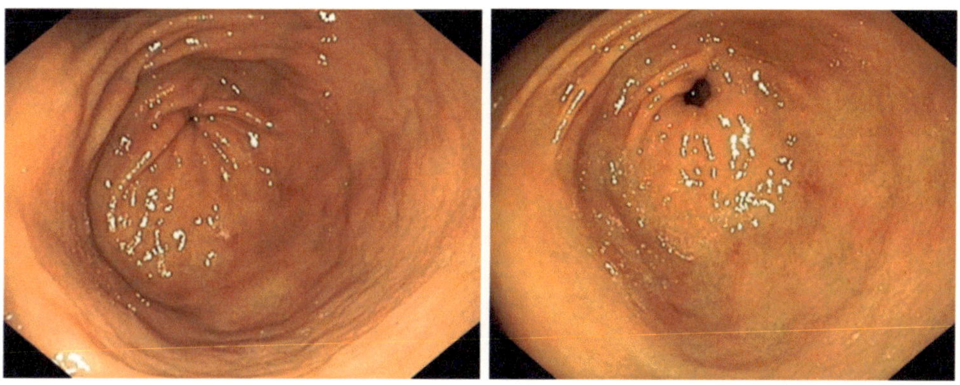

Figure 14.
Stomach: Helicobacter pylori *(negative) and CMV (positive).*

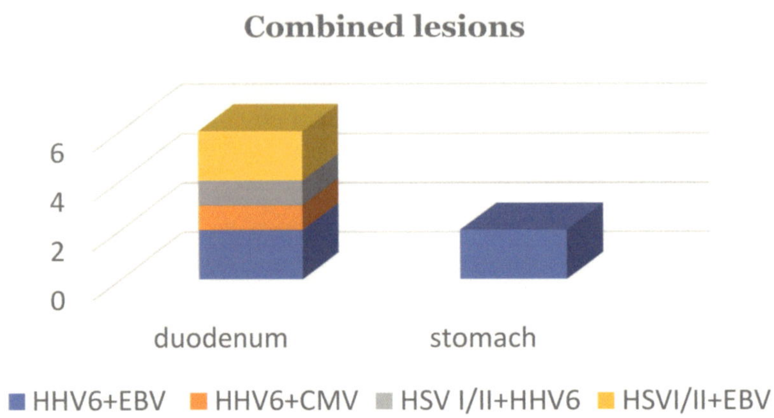

Figure 15.
Variants of combined lesions of the gastric and duodenal mucosa.

and 1.64%); HSV I/II + HHV6 in 1 patient (1.78 and 1.64%); and HSV I/II + EBV in 2 patients (3.57 and 3.27%). In gastric biopsies, combined HHV6 + EBV lesions were detected in 2 patients (40 and 3.27%).

Endoscopic images of some cases with combined herpes virus lesions of the mucous membranes of the stomach and duodenum are presented in **Figures 16–19** (from the archives of Dr. Umud Mahmudov).

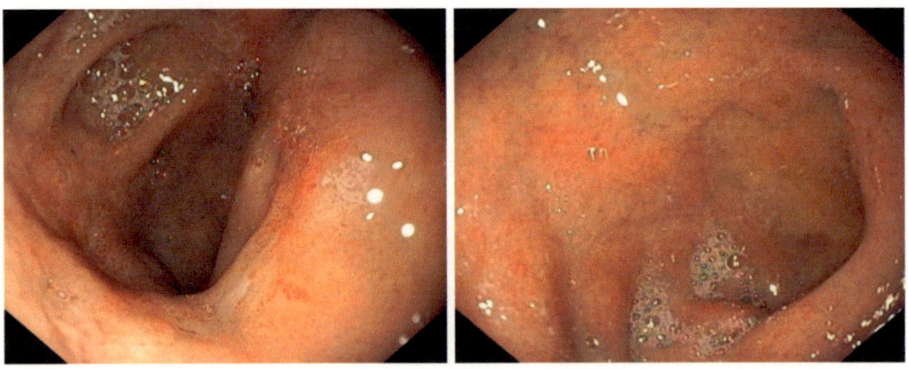

Figure 16.
Duodenum: Helicobacter pylori *(negative), HSV6 (positive) u CMV (positive).*

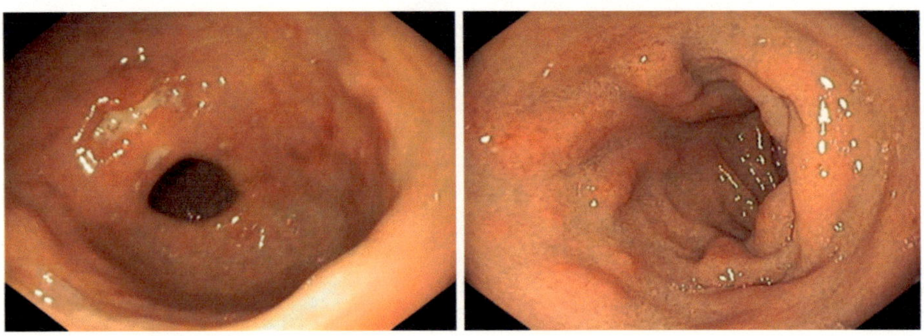

Figure 17.
Stomach and duodenum: Helicobacter pylori *(negative), HSV I (positive) u EBV (positive).*

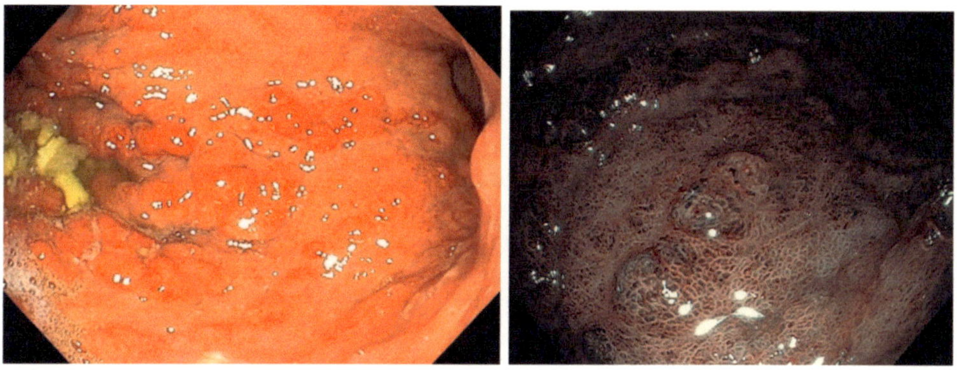

Figure 18.
Stomach: Helicobacter pylori *(negative) u HHV6 (positive).*

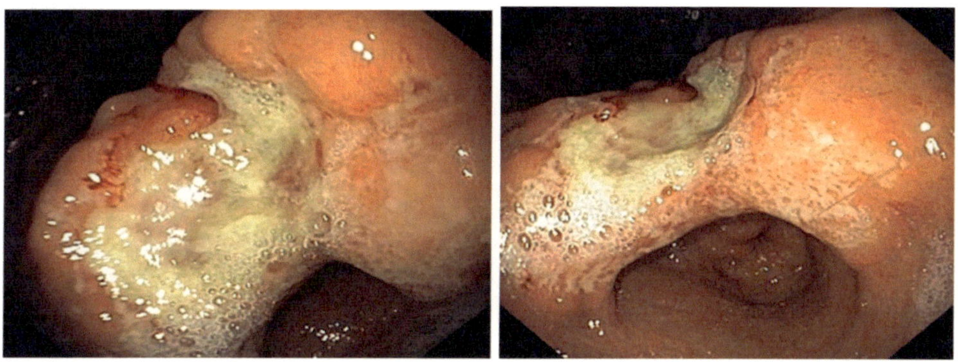

Figure 19.
Stomach: Helicobacter pylori *(negative) u EBV (positive).*

Thus, the conclusions we came to as a result of our research are:

The incidence of herpesviruses in patients with successful eradication of *H. pylori* but with preserved clinical complaints was 68.5%. Given the problems and frequency of malignancy in this part of the digestive tract, more attention should be paid to this problem.

A definite relationship was found between the identified herpes viruses and changes during endoscopic and morphological searches. So, for ulcerative lesions, the detection of CMV and HSV I/II ($p = 0.009$) was more typical, for changes in the architectonics of duodenal villi - EBV ($p=0.008$), for polyps - HHV6 ($p = 0.009$).

If the patient's complaints continue after the positive eradication of *H. pylori*, and mucosal damage is visible in the endoscopic image, we recommend PCR examination of herpes viruses from the tissue.

For ulcerative lesions, the detection of CMV and HSV I/II was more typical, for changes in the architectonics of duodenal villi - EBV, for polyps - HHV6.

Given the large-scale epidemiological and clinical significance of *Helicobacter pylori* as an infectious agent with high oncogenic potential, as well as its ability to affect not only the gastrointestinal tract but also to have a systemic effect beyond the digestive system, the problem of timely diagnosis and effective eradication therapy remains extremely relevant. Particular attention is paid to the issues of choosing treatment regimens for both the first line and subsequent lines, with the need to adapt them depending on regional characteristics of the prevalence of resistant strains, age categories of patients, and the availability of therapy. These aspects are actively discussed both at the level of the European scientific community [98–102] and in the context of national data, including the situation in our country [103, 104]. Against this background, the simultaneous presence of herpes viruses in the body, in particular the Epstein-Barr virus and cytomegalovirus, which can persist and reactivate in the mucous membrane of the stomach and duodenum, brings to the fore new aspects of pathogenesis, diagnostics, and patient management tactics. There is a need for a comprehensive approach that takes into account not only the presence of *H. pylori* but also potential coinfection with herpes viruses, especially in patients with chronic gastritis, peptic ulcer disease, and neoplastic processes.

Thus, new realities require expanded clinical and diagnostic thinking, including molecular screening and immunoassessment, for the timely detection of coinfections and selection of individualized, pathogenetically substantiated therapy. Integration of these data into clinical practice can significantly improve the effectiveness of prevention and treatment of upper gastrointestinal diseases, as well as reduce the risks of progression to precancerous and malignant conditions.

13. Conclusion

The question of the nature of the interaction between *Helicobacter pylori* and human herpesviruses—in particular, Epstein-Barr virus (EBV) and cytomegalovirus (CMV)—in the pathogenesis of diseases of the stomach and duodenum remains open and requires further study. Modern data demonstrate both the potential synergy of these pathogens and their ability to cause pathological changes independently of each other. On the one hand, *H. pylori*, EBV, and CMV have the ability to cause chronic inflammation, modulate the host immune response, and induce epigenetic changes, creating a favorable environment for cell transformation. Their coinfection can increase tissue damage, activate cross-signaling pathways (NF-κB, MAPK, WNT/β-catenin, etc.), and increase the risk of oncogenesis. A number of studies indicate an increased prevalence of viral infections in the presence of *H. pylori*, as well as a more severe course of gastritis and peptic ulcer disease in coinfection, especially in predisposed individuals.

On the other hand, each of these pathogens is capable of causing inflammatory and neoplastic processes independently, which is confirmed by cases of gastric cancer and peptic ulcer disease in patients with isolated infection with either *H. pylori* or EBV/CMV. In addition, a competitive scenario is possible, in which one of the agents suppresses the activity of the other through immunomodulatory mechanisms.

Thus, at the current stage of scientific development, there is no clear answer to the question: do *H. pylori* and herpesviruses act as "accomplices" in the pathogenesis of gastrointestinal diseases, or as "independent players"? Most likely, both models are possible depending on the individual characteristics of the patient, immune status, virulence of strains, and duration of infection.

Given the potential significance of coinfection for clinical practice, it seems important not only to identify each of these pathogens in the diagnosis of diseases of the stomach and duodenum but also to analyze their possible interactions. Further molecular epidemiological studies are needed to better understand the mechanism of their joint or separate participation in the pathogenesis and progression of benign and malignant diseases of the gastrointestinal tract.

Author details

Gulustan H. Babayeva[1,2*], Umud R. Mahmudov[3], Jamal S. Musayev[4], Ferid V. Guliyev[5], Emin Kh. Verdiyev[6], Rashad A. Hasanov[1,7], Gunay V. Asadova[1,5], Rafail H. Hasanov[8], Aychin I. Hasanova[1] and Nargiz E. Afandiyeva[5]

1 Department of Therapy, Azerbaijan State Advanced Training Institute for Doctors Named after A. Alıyev, Baku, Azerbaijan

2 Memorial Hospital, Baku, Azerbaijan

3 Department of Gastroenterology and Endoscopy, Modern Hospital, Baku, Azerbaijan

4 Baku Pathology Center, Pathomorphology Department, Baku, Azerbaijan

5 National Centre of Oncology, Department of Invasive Diagnosis and Treatment, Baku, Azerbaijan

6 Department of Gastroenterology and Endoscopy, Central Hospital, Baku, Azerbaijan

7 Department of Gastroenterology and Endoscopy, German Hospital, Baku, Azerbaijan

8 Diaqnoz Medical Center, Department of Gastroenterology and Endoscopy, Baku, Azerbaijan

*Address all correspondence to: ghbabayeva@gmail.com

References

[1] Strzelczyk JK, Świętek A, Hudy D, Gołąbek K, Gaździcka J, Miśkiewicz-Orczyk K, et al. Low prevalence of HSV-1 and helicobacter pylori in HNSCC and chronic tonsillitis patients compared to healthy individuals. Diagnostics. 2023;**13**(10):1798. DOI: 10.3390/diagnostics13101798

[2] Jain M. Assesment of correlation of herpes simplex virus-1 with oral cancer and precancer-a comparative study. Journal of Clinical and Diagnostic Research. 2016;**10**:ZC14-ZC17

[3] Packard JE, Dembowski JA. HSV-1 DNA replication—Coordinated regulation by viral and cellular factors. Viruses. 2021;**13**:2015

[4] Starr JR, Daling JR, Fitzgibbons ED, Madeleine MM, Ashley R, Galloway DA, et al. Serologic evidence of herpes simplex virus 1 infection and oropharyngeal cancer risk. Cancer Research. 2001;**61**:8459-8464

[5] Looker KJ, Magaret AS, May MT, Turner KM, Vickerman P, Gottlieb SL, et al. Global and regional estimates of prevalent and incident herpes simplex virus type 1 infections in 2012. PLoS One. 2015;**10**:e0140765

[6] Arshad Z, Alturkistani A, Brindley D, Lam C, Foley K, Meinert E. Tools for the diagnosis of herpes simplex virus 1/2: Systematic review of studies published between 2012 and 2018. JMIR Public Health and Surveillance. 2019;**5**:e14216

[7] Ramchandani M, Kong M, Tronstein E, Selke S, Mikhaylova A, Magaret A, et al. Herpes simplex virus type 1 shedding in tears and nasal and oral mucosa of healthy adults. Sexually Transmitted Diseases. 2016;**43**:756-760

[8] Krasteva A, Petrova M. Dualistic face of H. pylori and some herpes viruses co-infection observation from clinical practice. The Journal of Gastroenterology and Hepatology Open Access. 2017;**6**(4):00204. DOI: 10.15406/ghoa.2017.06.00204

[9] Balfour HH, Sifakis F, Sliman JA, et al. Age-specific prevalence of Epstein-Barr virus infection among individuals aged 6-19 years in the United States and factors affecting its acquisition. The Journal of Infectious Diseases. 2013;**208**(8):1286-1293

[10] Hsu JL, Glaser SL. Epstein-Barr virus-associated malignancies: Epidemiologic patterns and etiologic implications. Critical Reviews in Oncology/Hematology. 2000;**34**(1):27-53

[11] Wang C, Liu Y, Xu LT, et al. Effects of ag-ing, cytomegalovirus infection, and EBV infection on human B cell repertoires. Journal of Immunology. 2014;**192**(2):603-611

[12] Petrova M, Kamburov V. Epstein-Barr virus: Silent companion or causative agent of chronic liver disease? World Journal of Gastroenterology. 2010;**16**(33):4130-4134

[13] Hasni SA. Role of Helicobacter pylori infection in autoimmune diseases. Current Opinion in Rheumatology. 2012;**24**(4):429-434

[14] Tsamakidis K, Panotopoulou E, Dimitroulopoulos D, et al. Herpes simplex virus type 1 in peptic ulcer disease: An inverse association with helicobacter pylori. World Journal of Gastroenterology. 2005;**11**(42):6644-6649

[15] Baccaglini L, Schoenbach VJ, Poole C, et al. Association between herpes simplex virus type 1 and Helicobacter pylori in US adolescents. Oral Surgery, Oral Medicine, Oral Pathology, Oral Radiology, and Endodontics. 2016;**101**(1):63-69

[16] Fuentes-Pananá EM, Morales-Sánchez A. Epstein-Barr virus-associated gastric cancer and potential mechanisms of oncogenesis. Current Cancer Drug Targets. 2017;**17**(6):534-554. DOI: 10.2174/1568009616666160926124923

[17] Saju P, Murata-Kamiya N, Hayashi T, et al. Host SHP1 phosphatase antagonizes Helicobacter pylori CagA and can be downregulated by Epstein-Barr virus. Nature Microbiology. 2016;**14**(1):16026

[18] Wu WK, Yu J, Chan MT, et al. Combinatorial epigenetic deregulation by He-licobacter pylori and Epstein-Barr virus infections in gastric tumourigenesis. The Journal of Pathology. 2016;**239**(3):245-249

[19] Cárdenas-Mondragón MG, Torres J, Flores-Luna L, et al. Epstein-Barr virus association with peptic ulcer disease. Analytical Cellular Pathology (Amsterdam). 2015;**2015**:164840

[20] Cárdenas-Mondragón MG, Torres J, Flores-Luna L, et al. Case–control study of Epstein–Barr virus and Helicobacter pylori serology in Latin American patients with gastric disease. British Journal of Cancer. 2015;**112**(12):1866-1873

[21] Singh S, Jha HC. Status of Epstein-Barr virus coinfection with Helicobacter pylori in gastric cancer. Journal of Oncology. 2017;**2017**:3456264. DOI: 10.1155/2017/3456264. Epub 2017 Mar 21

[22] Ferrasi AC, Pinheiro NA, Rabenhorst SHB, et al. Helicobacter pylori and EBV in gastric carcinomas: Methylation status and microsatellite instability. World Journal of Gastroenterology. 2010;**16**(3):312-319. DOI: 10.3748/wjg.v16.i3.312

[23] Minoura-Etoh J, Gotoh K, Sato R, et al. Helicobacter pylori-associated oxidant monochloramine induces reactivation of Epstein-Barr virus (EBV) in gastric epithelial cells latently infected with EBV. Journal of Medical Microbiology. 2006;**55**(part 7):905-911. DOI: 10.1099/jmm.0.46580-0

[24] Shukla SK, Prasad KN, Tripathi A, et al. Epstein-Barr virus DNA load and its association with Helicobacter pylori infection in gastroduodenal diseases. Brazilian Journal of Infectious Diseases. 2011;**15**(6):583-590. DOI: 10.1016/s1413-8670(11)70255-0

[25] Cárdenas-Mondragón MG, Carreón-Talavera R, Camorlinga-Ponce M, Gomez-Delgado A, Torres J, Fuentes-Pananá EM. Epstein barr virus and Helicobacter pylori co-infection are positively associated with severe gastritis in pediatric patients. PLoS One. 2013;**8**(4):e62850. DOI: 10.1371/journal.pone.0062850.e62850

[26] Martínez-Carrillo DN, Atrisco-Morales J, Hernández-Pando R, et al. Helicobacter pylori vacA and cagA genotype diversity and interferon gamma expression in patients with chronic gastritis and patients with gastric cancer. Revista de Gastroenterologia de Mexico. 2014;**79**(4):220-228. DOI: 10.1016/j.rgmx.2014.10.003

[27] Noach LA, Bosma NB, Jansen J, Hoek FJ, van Deventer SJH, Tytgat GNJ. Mucosal tumor necrosis factor-or, interleukin-1/3, and interleukin-8 production in patients with helicobacter pylori infection. Scandinavian Journal of Gastroenterology. 1994;**29**(5):425-429. DOI: 10.3109/00365529409096833

[28] Yamaoka Y, Kita M, Kodama T, Sawai N, Imanishi J. Helicobacter pylori cagA gene and expression of cytokine messenger RNA in gastric mucosa. Gastroenterology. 1996;**110**(6):1744-1752. DOI: 10.1053/gast.1996.v110.pm8964399

[29] El-Omar EM, Rabkin CS, Gammon MD, et al. Increased risk of noncardia gastric cancer associated with proinflammatory cytokine gene polymorphisms. Gastroenterology. 2003;**124**(5):1193-1201. DOI: 10.1016/S0016-5085(03)00157-4

[30] Churin Y, Al-Ghoul L, Kepp O, Meyer TF, Birchmeier W, Naumann M. Helicobacter pylori CagA protein targets the c-met receptor and enhances the motogenic response. Journal of Cell Biology. 2003;**161**(2):249-255. DOI: 10.1083/jcb.200208039

[31] Brandt S, Wessler S, Hartig R, Backert S. Helicobacter pylori activates protein kinase C delta to control Raf in MAP kinase signalling: Role in AGS epithelial cell scattering and elongation. Cell Motility and the Cytoskeleton. 2009;**66**(10):874-892. DOI: 10.1002/cm.20373

[32] Ohnishi N, Yuasa H, Tanaka S, et al. Transgenic expression of helicobacter pylori CagA induces gastrointestinal and hematopoietic neoplasms in mouse. Proceedings of the National Academy of Sciences of the United States of America. 2008;**105**(3):1003-1008. DOI: 10.1073/pnas.0711183105

[33] Miura M, Ohnishi N, Tanaka S, Yanagiya K, Hatakeyama M. Differential oncogenic potential of geographically distinct helicobacter pylori CagA isoforms in mice. International Journal of Cancer. 2009;**125**(11):2497-2504. DOI: 10.1002/ijc.24740

[34] Kaplan-Türköz B, Jiménez-Soto LF, Dian C, et al. Structural insights into Helicobacter pylori oncoprotein CagA interaction with β1 integrin. Proceedings of the National Academy of Sciences of the United States of America. 2012;**109**(36):14640-14645. DOI: 10.1073/pnas.1206098109

[35] Nešić D, Buti L, Lu X, Stebbins CE. Structure of the Helicobacter pylori CagA oncoprotein bound to the human tumor suppressor ASPP2. Proceedings of the National Academy of Sciences of the United States of America. 2014;**111**(4):1562-1567. DOI: 10.1073/pnas.1320631111

[36] Dawson CW, Port RJ, Young LS. The role of the EBV-encoded latent membrane proteins LMP1 and LMP2 in the pathogenesis of nasopharyngeal carcinoma (NPC). Seminars in Cancer Biology. 2012;**22**(2):144-153. DOI: 10.1016/j.semcancer.2012.01.004

[37] Tegtmeyer N, Wessler S, Backert S. Role of the cag-pathogenicity island encoded type IV secretion system in Helicobacter pylori pathogenesis. The FEBS Journal. 2011;**278**(8):1190-1202. DOI: 10.1111/j.1742-4658.2011.08035.x

[38] Neal JT, Peterson TS, Kent ML, Guillemin KH. Pylori virulence factor CagA increases intestinal cell proliferation by Wnt pathway activation in a transgenic zebrafish model. Disease Models and Mechanisms. 2013;**6**(3):802-810. DOI: 10.1242/dmm.011163

[39] Pilon N, Oh K, Sylvestre J-R, Savory JGA, Lohnes D. Wnt signaling is a key mediator of Cdx1 expression in vivo. Development. 2007;**134**(12):2315-2323. DOI: 10.1242/dev.001206

[40] Fujii Y, Yoshihashi K, Suzuki H, et al. CDX1 confers intestinal phenotype on gastric epithelial cells via induction of stemness-associated reprogramming factors SALL4 and KLF5. Proceedings

of the National Academy of Sciences of the United States of America. 2012;**109**(50):20584-20589. DOI: 10.1073/pnas.1208651109

[41] Yu X-W, Xu Y, Gong Y-H, Qian X, Yuan Y. Helicobacter pylori induces malignant transformation of gastric epithelial cells in vitro. APMIS. 2011;**119**(3):187-197. DOI: 10.1111/j.1600-0463.2010.02709.x

[42] Szkaradkiewicz A, Karpiński TM, Majewski J, Malinowska K, Goślińska-Kuźniarek O, Linke K. The participation of p53 and bcl-2 proteins in gastric carcinomas associated with helicobacter pylori and/or Epstein-Barr virus (EBV). Polish Journal of Microbiology. 2015;**64**(3):211-216

[43] Yu J, Cheng YY, Tao Q, et al. Methylation of protocadherin 10, a novel tumor suppressor, is associated with poor prognosis in patients with gastric cancer. Gastroenterology. 2009;**136**(2):640-651.e1. DOI: 10.1053/j.gastro.2008.10.050

[44] Pimson C, Ekalaksananan T, Pientong C, et al. Aberrant methylation of PCDH10 and RASSF1A genes in blood samples for non-invasive diagnosis and prognostic assessment of gastric cancer. PeerJ. 2016;**4**:e2112. DOI: 10.7717/peerj.2112.e2112

[45] Schneider BG, Piazuelo MB, Sicinschi LA, et al. Virulence of infecting Helicobacter pylori strains and intensity of mononuclear cell infiltration are associated with levels of DNA hypermethylation in gastric mucosae. Epigenetics. 2013;**8**(11):1153-1161. DOI: 10.4161/epi.26072

[46] Wu WKK, Yu J, Chan MTV, To K. F, Cheng ASL. Combinatorial epigenetic deregulation by Helicobacter pylori and Epstein–Barr virus infections in gastric tumourigenesis. Journal of Pathology. 2016;**239**(3):245-249. DOI: 10.1002/path.4731

[47] Saju P, Murata-Kamiya N, Hayashi T, et al. Host SHP1 phosphatase antagonizes Helicobacter pyloriCagA and can be downregulated by Epstein-Barr virus. Nature Microbiology. 2016;**1**(4):16026. DOI: 10.1038/nmicrobiol.2016.26.16026

[48] Buzás GM, Konderák J. Co-infection with helicobacter pylori and Epstein-Barr virus in benign upper digestive diseases: An endoscopic and serologic pilot study. United European Gastroenterology Journal. 2016;**4**(3):388-394. DOI: 10.1177/2050640615610265

[49] Shukla SK, Khatoon J, Prasad KN, et al. Transforming growth factor beta 1 (TGF-β1) modulates Epstein-Barr virus reactivation in absence of Helicobacter pylori infection in patients with gastric cancer. Cytokine. 2016;**77**:176-179. DOI: 10.1016/j.cyto.2015.07.023

[50] Ong DS, Spitoni C, Klein Klouwenberg P, Verduyn Lunel FM, Frencken JF, Schultz MJ, et al. Cytomegalovirus reactivation and mortality in patients with acute respiratory distress syndrome. Intensive Care Medicine. 2016;**42**:333-341

[51] Wills MR, Poole E, Lau B, Krishna B, Sinclair JH. The immunology of human cytomegalovirus latency: Could latent infection be cleared by novel immunotherapeutic strategies? Cellular and Molecular Immunology. 2015;**12**:128-138

[52] Allah HAZ, Obayes AL-KFH, Obayes A-HAD, Mahdi ARS. Correlation between H. Pylori and cytomegalovirus in adults. Medical Journal of Dr. D.Y. Patil Vidyapeeth. 2024;**17**(1):106-109. DOI: 10.4103/mjdrdypu.mjdrdypu_615_22

[53] Zamani M, Ebrahimtabar F, Zamani V, Miller WH, Alizadeh-Navaei R, Shokri-Shirvani J, et al. Systematic review with meta-analysis: The worldwide prevalence of Helicobacter pylori infection. Alimentary Pharmacology and Therapeutics. 2018;**47**:868-876

[54] Thung I, Aramin H, Vavinskaya V, Gupta S, Park JY, Crowe SE, et al. The global emergence of helicobacter pylori antibiotic resistance. Alimentary Pharmacology and Therapeutics. 2016;**43**:514-533

[55] Al-Khikani FH. Dermatophytosis a worldwide contiguous fungal infection: Growing challenge and few solutions. Biomedical And Biotechnology Research Journal. 2020;**4**:117

[56] Al-Khikani FH, Almosawey HA, Abdullah YJ, Al-Asadi AA, Hameed RM, Hasan NF, et al. Potential antiviral properties of antifungal drugs. The Journal of The Egyptian Women's Dermatologic Society. 2020;**17**:185

[57] O'Connor A, O'Moráin C. Helicobacter pylori infection in Europe: Current perspectives. Expert Review of Gastroenterology and Hepatology. 2013;**7**:541-548

[58] Krueger W, Hilborn E, Converse R, Wade T. Environmental risk factors associated with Helicobacter pylori seroprevalence in the United States: A cross-sectional analysis of NHANES data. Epidemiology and Infection. 2015;**143**:2520-2531

[59] Inoue M. Changing epidemiology of Helicobacter pylori in Japan. Gastric Cancer. 2017;**20**:3-7

[60] Eshraghian A. Epidemiology of Helicobacter pylori infection among the healthy population in Iran and countries of the eastern Mediterranean region: A systematic review of prevalence and risk factors. World Journal of Gastroenterology. 2014;**20**:17618-17625

[61] Del Moral-Hernández O, Castañón-Sánchez CA, Reyes-Navarrete S, Martínez-Carrillo DN, Betancourt-Linares R, Jiménez-Wences H, et al. Multiple infections by EBV, HCMV and Helicobacter pylori are highly frequent in patients with chronic gastritis and gastric cancer from Southwest Mexico: An observational study. Medicine. 2019;**98**:37

[62] Chen C, Chen S, Han Z, Xie W, Zhang T, Mao C, et al. Patients with helicobacter pylori-positive gastric cancer with human cytomegalovirus infection have a low tendency of advanced lymphatic metastasis in a Chinese population. Oncology Letters. 2021;**21**:1-9

[63] Yoo Y, Lee Y, Lee YM, Choe YH. Co-infection with cytomegalovirus and Helicobacter pylori in a child with Ménétrier's disease. Pediatric Gastroenterology, Hepatology and Nutrition. 2013;**16**:123-126

[64] Kreidieh M, Gurala D, Amarnath S, Philipose J, Colef R, Yassine AA, et al. The unmasking of cytomegalovirus as an accomplice to Helicobacter pylori–induced severe acute gastroenteritis in a healthy host. ACG Case Reports Journal. 2023;**10**(10):e01181. DOI: 10.14309/crj.0000000000001181

[65] Taylor GH. American Family Physician. 2003;**67**(3):519-524

[66] Jain M, Duggal S, Chugh TD. Cytomegalovirus infection in non-immunosuppressed critically ill patients. Journal of Infection in Developing Countries. 2011;**5**(08):571-579

[67] Ahmed A. Antiviral treatment of cytomegalovirus infection.

Infectious Disorders Drug Targets. 2011;**11**(5):475-503

[68] Bencharif L, Cathébras P, Bouchou K, Gouilloud S, Fichtner C, Rousset H. Exudative gastroenteropathy revealing primary CMV infection in an immunocompetent adult. La Revue de Médecine Interne. 1998;**19**:288-290

[69] Chetty R, Roskell DE. Cytomegalovirus infection in the gastrointestinal tract. Journal of Clinical Pathology. 1994;**47**(11):968-972

[70] Sinclair J, Sissons P. Latency and reactivation of human cytomegalovirus. The Journal of General Virology. 2006;**87**(7):1763-1779

[71] Crough T, Khanna R. Immunobiology of human cytomegalovirus: From bench to bedside. Clinical Microbiology Reviews. 2009;**22**(1):76-98

[72] Jackson SE, Mason GM, Wills MR. Human cytomegalovirus immunity and immune evasion. Virus Research. 2011;**157**(2):151-160

[73] Rafailidis PI, Mourtzoukou EG, Varbobitis IC, Falagas ME. Severe cytomegalovirus infection in apparently immunocompetent patients: A systematic review. Virology Journal. 2008;**5**(1):47

[74] Hulo P, Touchefeu Y, Cauchin E, et al. Acute ulceronecrotic gastritis with cytomegalovirus reactivation: Uncommon toxicity of immune checkpoint inhibitors in microsatellite instability-high metastatic colorectal cancer. Clinical Colorectal Cancer. 2020;**19**(4):e183-e188

[75] Nikolich-Žugich J, Čicin-Šain L, Collins-McMillen D, et al. Advances in cytomegalovirus (CMV) biology and its relationship to health, diseases, and aging. Geroscience. 2020;**42**(2):495-504

[76] Li W, Fan H, Yiping L. Postural epigastric pain as a sign of cytomegalovirus gastritis in renal transplant recipients: A case-based review. Transplantation Proceedings. 2009;**41**(9):3956-3958

[77] Gravito-Soares E, Almeida N. Cytomegalovirus disease of the upper gastrointestinal tract: An emerging infection in immunocompetent hosts. GE Portuguese Journal of Gastroenterology. 2017;**24**(6):259-261

[78] Gökçe Ş, Kurugöl Z. Cytomegalovirus-associated menetrier disease in childhood. Clinical Pediatrics (Phila). 2017;**56**(4):382-384

[79] Canan O, Ozçay F, Bilezikçi B. Ménétrier's disease and severe gastric ulcers associated with cytomegalovirus infection in an immunocompetent child: A case report. The Turkish Journal of Pediatrics. 2008;**50**(3):291-295

[80] Ljungman P, Griffiths P, Paya C. Definitions of cytomegalovirus infection and disease in transplant recipients. Clinical Infectious Diseases. 2002;**34**(8):1094-1097

[81] Maiorana A, Baccarini P, Foroni M, Bellini N, Giusti F. Human cytomegalovirus infection of the gastrointestinal tract in apparently immunocompetent patients. Human Pathology. 2003;**34**(12):1331-1336

[82] Ebisutani C, Kawamura A, Shibata N, et al. Gastric ulcer associated with cytomegalovirus in an immunocompetent patient: Method for diagnosis. Case Reports in Gastroenterology. 2012;**6**(2):365-368

[83] Rich A, Toro TZ, Tanksley J, et al. Distinguishing Ménétrier's disease from its mimics. Gut. 2010;**59**(12):1617-1624

[84] Lin WR, Su MY, Hsu CM, et al. Clinical and endoscopic features for alimentary tract cytomegalovirus disease: Report of 20 cases with gastrointestinal cytomegalovirus disease. Chang Gung Medical Journal. 2005;**28**(7):476-484

[85] Reggiani Bonetti L, Losi L, Di Gregorio C, et al. Cytomegalovirus infection of the upper gastrointestinal tract: A clinical and pathological study of 30 cases. Scandinavian Journal of Gastroenterology. 2011;**46**(10):1228-1235

[86] Himoto T, Goda F, Okuyama H, et al. Cytomegalovirus-associated acute gastric mucosal lesion in an immunocompetent host. Internal Medicine. 2009;**48**(17):1521-1524

[87] Gandhi MK, Khanna R. Human cytomegalovirus: Clinical aspects, immune regulation, and emerging treatments. The Lancet Infectious Diseases. 2004;**4**(12):725-738

[88] Jang EY, Park S, Lee E, et al. Diagnostic performance of the cytomegalovirus (CMV) antigenemia assay in patients with CMV gastrointestinal disease. Clinical Infectious Diseases. 2009;**48**(12):e121-e124

[89] Graham DY, Opekun AR, Yamaoka Y, Osato MS, El-Zimaity HMT. Early events in proton pump inhibitor-associated exacerbation of corpus gastritis. Alimentary Pharmacology and Therapeutics. 2003;**17**(2):193-200

[90] Genta RM. Where have all the helicobacters gone? Journal of Clinical Gastroenterology. 2007;**41**(8):727-728

[91] Genta RM, Graham DY. Comparison of biopsy sites for the histopathologic diagnosis of Helicobacter pylori: A topographic study of H. pylori density and distribution. Gastrointestinal Endoscopy. 1994;**40**(3):342-345

[92] Tokuhara D, Okano Y, Asou K, Tamamori A, Yamano T. Cytomegalovirus and helicobacter pylori co-infection in a child with Ménétrier disease. European Journal of Pediatrics. 2006;**166**(1):63-65

[93] Ueno M, Shimodate Y, Yamamoto S, Yamamoto H, Mizuno M. Gastric cancer associated with refractory cytomegalovirus gastritis. Clinical Journal of Gastroenterology. 2017;**10**(6):498-502

[94] Del Moral-Hernández O, Castañón-Sánchez CA, Reyes-Navarrete S, et al. Multiple infections by EBV, HCMV and helicobacter pylori are highly frequent in patients with chronic gastritis and gastric cancer from Southwest Mexico: An observational study. Medicine (Baltimore). 2019;**98**(3):e14124

[95] Lv Y, Fei-fei H, Zhuo-ling A, et al. Cytomegalovirus infection is a risk factor in gastrointestinal cancer: A cross-sectional and meta-analysis study. Intervirology. 2020;**63**(1-6):10-16

[96] Malfertheiner P et al. Management of Helicobacter pylori infection Maastricht V/Florence consensus report. Gut. 2017;**66**(1):6-30

[97] Malfertheiner P, Megraud F, Rokkas T, et al. Gut. 2022;**71**:1724-1762. DOI: 10.1136/gutjnl-2022-327745

[98] García-Morales N, Pérez-Aisa A, Fiorini G, Tepes B, Castro-Fernández M, Lucendo AJ, et al. On behalf of the Hp-EuReg investigators. Helicobacter pylori diagnostic tests used in Europe: Results of over 34,000 patients from the European registry on helicobacter pylori management. Journal of Clinical Medicine. 2023;**12**(13):4363. DOI: 10.3390/jcm12134363

[99] Jonaitis P, Nyssen OP, Saracino IM, Fiorini G, Vaira D, Pérez-Aísa Á, et al. Comparison of the management of Helicobacter pylori infection between the older and younger European populations. Scientific Reports. 2023;**13**(1):17235. DOI: 10.1038/s41598-023-43287-4

[100] Olmedo L, Calvet X, Gené E, Bordin DS, Voynovan I, Castro-Fernandez M, et al. Evolution of the use, effectiveness and safety of bismuth-containing quadruple therapy for Helicobacter pylori infection between 2013 and 2021: Results from the European registry on H. pylori management (Hp-EuReg). Gut. 2024;**74**(1):15-25. DOI: 10.1136/gutjnl-2024-332804

[101] Huguet JM, Ferrer-Barceló L, Suárez P, Barcelo-Cerda S, Sempere J, Saracino IM, et al. Hp-EuReg investigators. Role of compliance in Helicobacter pylori eradication treatment: Results of the European registry on H. pylori management. United European. Gastroenterologisches Journal. 2024;**12**(6):691-704. DOI: 10.1002/ueg2.12569

[102] Martínez-Domínguez SJ, Nyssen OP, Lanas Á, Alfaro E, Jonaitis L, Mahmudov U, et al. Indications of helicobacter pylori eradication treatment and its influence on prescriptions and effectiveness (Hp-EuReg). Helicobacter. 2024;**29**(4):e13111. DOI: 10.1111/hel.13111

[103] Babayeva GH, Mahmudov UR, Mammadov EE, Guliyev FV, Verdiyev EK, Machanov UR, et al. First-line therapy prescriptions in Azerbaijan: Results from the European registry on Helicobacter pylori management (Hp-EuReg). Scientific-practical journal named after A.Aliyev "The Medicine and Science". 2024;**1**(35):55-65. Available from: https://n9.cl/oeo20

[104] Babayeva GH, Mahmudov UR, Mammadov EE, Guliyev FV, Verdiyev EK, Machanov UR, et al. Effectiveness of first-line empirical treatment in Azerbaijan: Results from the European registry on Helicobacter pylori management (Hp-EuReg). Scientific-Practical Journal Named after A.Aliyev "The Medicine and Science". 2024;**2**(36):34-47. Available from: https://n9.cl/tw7cw0